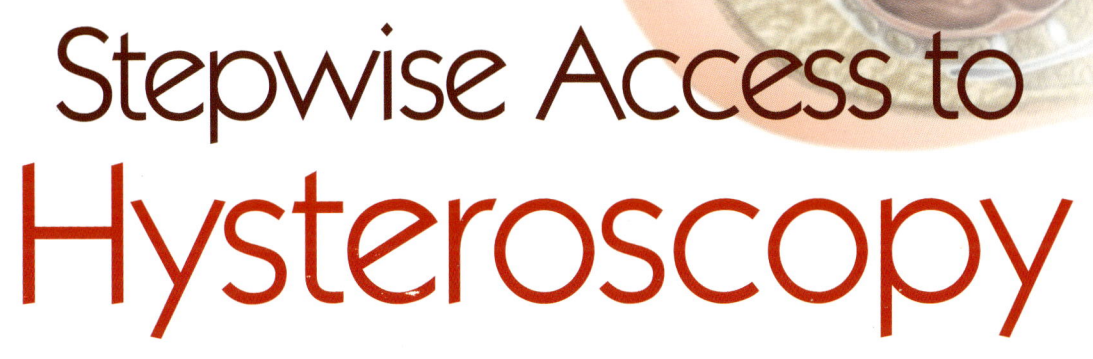

Stepwise Access to
Hysteroscopy

Stepwise Access to
Hysteroscopy

Richa Sharma MS, MNAMS, FICOG, FICMCH, FMAS

Associate Professor
Department of Obstetrics and Gynecology
University College of Medical Sciences and GTB Hospital
Delhi

email: gautamdrricha1@gmail.com

Rahul Manchanda MD, FICOG, FICMCH, FICS, FACS

Director
Manchanda's Endoscopic Center, New Delhi
Head, Gyne Endoscopy Unit, PSRI Hospital and Rosewalk Hospital
New Delhi
Founder Chairperson
International Hysteroscopy Congress

email: drrahulmanchanda@rediffmail.com

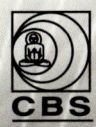

CBS

CBS Publishers & Distributors Pvt Ltd

New Delhi • Bengaluru • Chennai • Kochi • Kolkata • Mumbai
Bhopal • Bhubaneswar • Hyderabad • Jharkhand • Nagpur • Patna • Pune
• Uttarakhand • Dhaka (Bangladesh) • Kathmandu (Nepal)

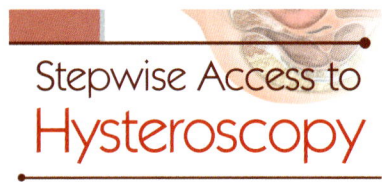

Stepwise Access to
Hysteroscopy

ISBN: 978-93-89688-53-5

Copyright © Authors and Publishers

First Edition: 2020

Published by Satish Kumar Jain and produced by Varun Jain for

CBS Publishers & Distributors Pvt Ltd
4819/XI Prahlad Street, 24 Ansari Road, Daryaganj, New Delhi 110 002, India.

Ph: 011-23289259, 23266861, 23266867   Fax: 011-23243014   Website: www.cbspd.com
e-mail: delhi@cbspd.com; cbspubs@airtelmail.in

Corporate Office: 204 FIE, Industrial Area, Patparganj, Delhi 110 092
Ph: 011-4934 4934   Fax: 011-4934 4935   e-mail: publishing@cbspd.com; publicity@cbspd.com

Branches

- **Bengaluru:** Seema House 2975, 17th Cross, K.R. Road, Banasankari 2nd Stage, Bengaluru 560 070, Karnataka
  Ph: +91-80-26771678/79   Fax: +91-80-26771680   e-mail: bangalore@cbspd.com
- **Chennai:** 7, Subbaraya Street, Shenoy Nagar, Chennai 600 030, Tamil Nadu
  Ph: +91-44-26260666, 26208620   Fax: +91-44-42032115   e-mail: chennai@cbspd.com
- **Kochi:** 68/1534, 35, 36 Power House Road, Opp. KSEB, Kochi 682018, Kerala
  Ph: +91-484-4059061-65   Fax: +91-484-4059065   e-mail: kochi@cbspd.com
- **Kolkata:** No. 6/B, Ground Floor, Rameswar Shaw Road, Kolkata 700014 (West Bengal), India
  Ph: +91-33-2289-1126, 2289-1127, 2289-1128   e-mail: kolkata@cbspd.com
- **Mumbai:** 83-C, Dr E Moses Road, Worli, Mumbai 400018, Maharashtra
  Ph: +91-22-24902340/41   Fax: +91-22-24902342   e-mail: mumbai@cbspd.com

Representatives

• **Bhopal**	0-8319310552	• **Bhubaneswar**	0-9911037372	• **Hyderabad**	0-9885175004
• **Jharkhand**	0-9811541605	• **Nagpur**	0-9421945513	• **Patna**	0-9334159340
• **Pune**	0-9623451994	• **Uttarakhand**	0-9716462459	• **Dhaka (Bangladesh)**	01912-003485
• **Kathmandu (Nepal)**	977-9818742655				

Printed at Nutech Print Services, Faridabad, India

Contributors

Aayushi Rathore MD
Senior Resident
Safdarjung Hospital
New Delhi

Alappat Kurian Joseph MD DGO
Director
Joseph Nursing Home/Hospital, Chennai, and
Board Member
International Society for Gynecologic Endoscopy
Member and AAGL
Chennai, India
numberdrkurian@gmail.com

Ashish Ramachandra Kale
MD, DNB, MNAMS, FICS, FICOG
Director
Ashakiran Hospitals and Asha IVF Center, Pune
Former Executive Vice President
Pune Obstetric and Gynecological Society
Managing Committee Member
IAGE and ISAR, Pune, India
drashishkale1978@yahoo.com

Fatema Ashraf FCPS, MPH (Epidemiology)
Professor and Head
Department of Obstetrics and Gynecology
Shaheed Suhrawardy Medical College
Dhaka, Bangladesh
fatema.phfbd2gmail.com

Gaetano Riemma MD
Consultant in Department of Women and Child
General and Specialized Surgery
University of Campania "Luigi Vaanvitelli" Naples
Italy
gaetanoriemma7@gmail.com

Giampietro Gubbini MD
Senior Consultent
Department of Gynecology
Madre Fortunata Toniolo Hospital, Bologna, Italy
ggubbini@gmail.com

Mario Franchini MD
Senior Consultent
Department of Gynecology
Regional Health Agency of Tuscany
Florence, Italy
framagi@alice.it

Mounir M Khalil MD
Specialist
Obstetrics and Gynecology
Endoscopic Surgeon
Cairo, Egypt
monisoft@gmail.com

PG Paul MD
Chairman
Paul's Hospital
Kaloor, Kochi
drpaulpg@gmail.com, paulshospital@gmail.com

Péter Török MD, PhD
Assistant Professor, Faculty of Medicine
Department of Obstetrics and Gynecology
University of Debrecen
Debrecen, Hungary
petertorokdr@gmail.com

Rahul Manchanda
MD, FICOG, FICMCH, FICS,FACS
Director
Manchanda's Endoscopic Center
New Delhi
Head
Gyne Endoscopy Unit
PSRI Hospital, New Delhi
drrahulmanchanda@rediff.com

Richa Sharma
MS, MNAMS,FICOG, FICMCH, FMAS
Associate Professor
Department of Obstetrics and Gynecology
University College of Medical Science and
GTB Hospital, Delhi
gautamdrricha1@gmail.com

Rokeya Begum MBBS, FCPS, MS
Adviser
University of Science and
Technology, Chittagong
Bangladesh
drrokeya_ctg@yahoo.com

Salvatore Giovanni Vitale MD, PhD
Senior Consultant
Unit of Gynecology and Obstetrics
Department of General Surgery, and
Medical Surgical Specialties
University of Catania, Italy
sgvitale@unict.it, vitalesalvatore@hotmail.com

Shahlagesmin MBBS, FCPS
Professor and Head
Department of Obstetrics and Gynecology
Rajshahi Medical College
Rajshahi, Bangladesh
shahelajessmin@gmail.com

Sushma Deshmukh MD, DGO
Director
Central India Test Tube Baby Centre
Head of the Department
Get Well Hospital and Research Institute
Nagpur

Foreword

The history of surgery is as old as the history of mankind. For centuries, man has tried to repair what was damaged in the human body. At first, it was considered an art, nowadays, it has become a scientific discipline, with a growing degree of sophistication.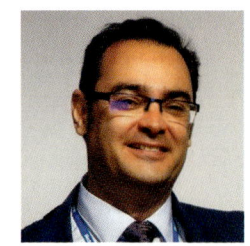

If three crucial periods were to be selected in the evolution of surgery, without a doubt, these are first, the invention of anesthesia; second, the antisepsis in the interventions; and third, the development of the minimally invasive surgery. These three facts have been a real turning point for surgery, regardless of the medical specialty which we refer to. All three were focused on improving both patient's safety and the outcome of the surgical procedure.

We can safely state that modern surgery started as such in 1846 at the Mass General Hospital in Boston, Massachusetts. It was there where anesthesia was used for the first time by aspiration of chemical gases during the surgical intervention. The patient was a young man diagnosed with tuberculosis with involvement of the tongue; the scheduled intervention: Removal of a maxillary tumor; and the surgeon was Dr John Collins Warren. This milestone in the history of medicine separated the excruciating suffering to which patients were subjected to during surgery and improved the way to apply the knowledge of so many surgeons around the world. Today, it would be unthinkable to perform certain interventions without the use of anesthesia.

The second moment that changed the history of surgery was the use of antisepsis. Post-surgical infections have been and continue to be one of the major problems of surgery. In the beginning, there were no minimum hygiene measures mandated during surgical procedures. It was Dr Semelweis, who introduced the recommendation of handwashing before interacting with patients. This extremely simple gesture had a tremendous impact in reducing the prevalence of infections related to wound manipulation. Before this intervention, it was thought that infections were spread by air and not by direct contact.

The third milestone is, without a doubt, the appearance of minimally invasive surgery. The development of gynecological endoscopy has meant a great advance in the accuracy of treatment of certain pathologies and in a better and faster recovery of the patients. Laparoscopy and hysteroscopy, both modalities in the fields of gynecologic surgery, have experienced in recent years an explosive advance, forcing us, gynecologic surgeons, to specialize and to keep up with a tremendous progress of technology.

Today hysteroscopy is experiencing a breakthrough. There are two fundamental reasons to explain this interesting momentum that hysteroscopy is having in modern gynecology. On the one hand, the development of new miniaturized instruments that favor a minimally invasive approach allowing the hysteroscopic treatment of a broad range of pathologies, thus increasing the indications of hysteroscopic surgery. The second reason is the increased interest in hysteroscopic surgery that gynecologists from all around the world have expressed embracing this amazing technology.

This change that has occurred in the world of hysteroscopy is forcing us to learn and to teach, looking for truthful and scientifically based sources of information and to innovate always basing our knowledge on truthful and solid scientific foundations. That is the purpose of this book: To compile in the different chapters that compose it, the most recent and up-to-date available information on the different topics that are here discussed. To create a guide, which helps everyone who enters their pages to improve their training as a gynecologic surgeon.

I will conclude with a recommendation, the degree of complexity of the instruments we use today, sometimes makes us behave more as health technicians than as doctors. Being a surgeon is not just operating well or using correctly all the devices we have in our operating room, but being a surgeon is a way to help others, is a way to solve problems or relieve pain, is to be part of the solution to the evils of others and is above all to apply common sense.

Being a surgeon is a lifestyle. Lets embrace it with pride!

Luis Alonso Pacheco
Medical Director, Reproductive Surgery Unit
Centro Gutenberg, Spain
Consultant, Reproductive Unit
Hospital Quirón Salud Malaga, Spain

Foreword

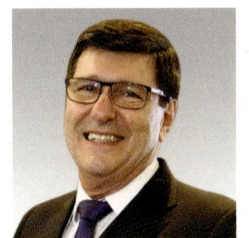

A hysteroscopic book has as its principles: A good orientation of the fundamentals, of the potential diagnostic of intrauterine diseases and surgical treatments, with operative techniques and appropriate technology. But, for this structure to represent correct information, the clinical staff must be of high technical knowledge and performance, expert in medical education, they must be teachers.

In this book, the reader will be able to obtain all these fundamentals, with an initial approach with presentation of instruments for out-patient procedures, such as, internal and external sheath, optics, graspers and scissors, for instruments for hospital procedures, such as resectoscope, morcellators, among others. Presenting the understanding of the necessary use of the distension medium with its different types, demonstrating its proper application, limits and risk of each one, so that everyone can perform ambulatory and hospital hysteroscopy with complete safety.

The discussion of operative techniques, with individualized and detailed description, including the most innovative and current technology, will lead us to a wide range of possibilities and options for performing the procedure.

The concern of the authors with the quality and depth of out-patient and hospital hysteroscopy is evident, through the description of the technique and new technology, risk and especially, the safety of the procedure, clearly identified by the selection of authors, known and recognized professors, as well as the placement of clinical cases to exemplify decisions and treatment possibilities.

Reading this work, with this quality, will interest those who are starting in hysteroscopy and those who already have experience in the method.

Congratulations to the authors and good reading to all.

Ricardo Bassil Lasmar
Professor
Associado de Ginecologia do
Departamento de Cirurgiae Especializada da
Universidade Federal Fluminense

Preface

This book is a comprehensive guide to hysteroscopy and provides all essential knowledge on basic and advanced hysteroscopy.

It gives information on procedure techniques, various innovations, clinical advances in practice and treatment of endometrial pathology.

The book is divided into two sections, Section I deals with all basic information like instrumentations, distension media, techniques of office hysteroscopy, complications, fluid deficit and monitoring and advanced hysteroscopy unit. Section II includes various case scenarios like cervical stenosis, hemorrhage, perforation, fluid overload and air embolism. Their preoperative and intraoperative precautions and management have been discussed in detail, along with suitable flowcharts, diagrams and algorithms for easy understanding of the contents.

The chapters have been discussed by the prominent experts in the field. Clearly formulated, organized and illustrated contents will enable the readers to gain maximum from each chapter.

This book will be a valuable source of knowledge to the gynecologists having keen interest in the field of hysteroscopy.

Richa Sharma
Rahul Manchanda

Acknowledgements

I express my deepest gratitude to all the eminent authors, who are from all over the world, for their valuable contribution of knowledge.

I am greatly thankful to Dr Rahul Manchanda, Director of Manchanda's Endoscopic Center and Head, Gyne Endoscopy Unit, PSRI Hospital, New Delhi, and also co-editor, for his expert guidance, support and encouragement.

I express my sincere thanks to Mr. Ramesh Krishnamachari, Regional Manager (Publishing), CBS Publishers & Distributors Pvt. Ltd, for his constant support and help in publishing this book.

I cannot express enough thanks to my loving and caring mother and daughter Gauri for providing immense support and motivation to accomplish this endeavor.

Richa Sharma

After the success of the first book, CBS Publishers requested and encouraged a second from the stables of MEC and IHC.

I must acknowledge all the co-authors who have given their time and experience so that this treatise could be produced. They are all friends and masters in their art and without them this would not have been possible.

Dr Richa, my colleague, worked tirelessly and endlessly shouldering the lions share of the work.

My mother has been my inspiration and has been my first teacher in the art of hysteroscopy and life. I thank her for always being there and holding my hand in my journey.

My wife Bhavna has unfailingly been by my side enduring my ungodly hours and erratic moods during my work. Thank you.

My girls Anya and Anvi who also have endured my moods, have given me the will to work and have kept me in good spirits and humor.

Finally, I thank my patients for providing me with the opportunity to look after them and gain knowledge and experience so I can share that for the greater good of women's health.

Rahul Manchanda

Contents

Section II   Different Case Scenarios

Management Algorithms: Diagnosis, Appropriate Preoperative Preparations and
Postoperative Management

Basic Knowledge on Hysteroscopy

Hysteroscopes: Equipment and Instruments, Hystero-optics and Vaginoscopic Technique

Mounir M Khalil

INTRODUCTION

The field of endoscopic surgery is a continuous cooperation between clinical knowledge, surgical skills, mechanical engineering and digital technologies.

The outcome of a procedure depends on the selection and specifications of the instruments involved and the surgeon's ability to use them in the right way. Contraindications of operations include unfamiliarity with the tools. For these reasons, it is always beneficial to invest some time and effort to have a brief overview on different tools involved in practice of hysteroscopy.

The Concept of Hysteroscopy

The female genital tract (vagina, cervix, uterine cavity and fallopian tubes) is a dark, collapsed, potential cavity. The main concept of any tool to visualize the interior of this cavity is to:
- Distend this cavity
- Light up the cavity
- Provide a means of acquiring the view from inside

To add an intervention, we need
- Access to an instrument
- Outflow to "wash out" the distension media.

The main challenge in hysteroscopy is that all the procedures have to be carried out through the only natural port, the uterine cervix (Fig. 1.1).

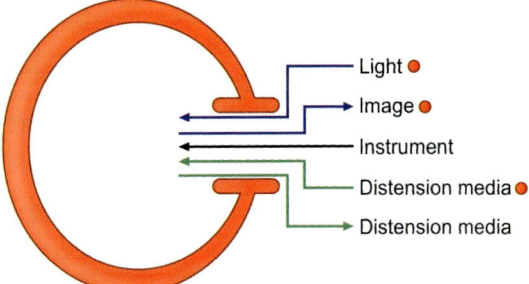

Fig. 1.1: The concept of hysteroscopy

Without cervical dilatation, the maximum caliber of the device should be 5 mm or less, and can be used without anesthesia (office based hysteroscopy), while with dilatation under anesthesia, cervix can reach 9 mm in diameter allowing larger devices to operate.

Because of the small diameters, we usually measure the tools in "French", rather than "millimeters", given that 1 mm = 3 Fr.

Design-wise, there are four categories of hysteroscopes now, namely
1. Diagnostic hysteroscopes
2. Operative hysteroscopes
3. Resectoscopes
4. Tissue removal systems

This chapter covers their types, structures, functions and differences between them, in addition to their usage and care, instructions along with their accessories.

Telescopes

The core piece of any endoscope is the telescope, it is the optical device that goes inside the organ cavity, transmits light from outside to inside and receives the image from inside to be seen from the other end outside.

Flexible telescopes (used with flexible hysteroscopes) are not widely used today due to their high cost, lower durability, limited functionality and sterilization inconvenience (Fig. 1.2).

Rigid telescopes are more common and standard. These are long metal cylinders housing some optic fibers for light transmission and a complex system of cylindrical lenses (Hopkins rod system) (Fig. 1.3).

Telescopes are available in many lengths, diameters and viewing angles. In hystero-

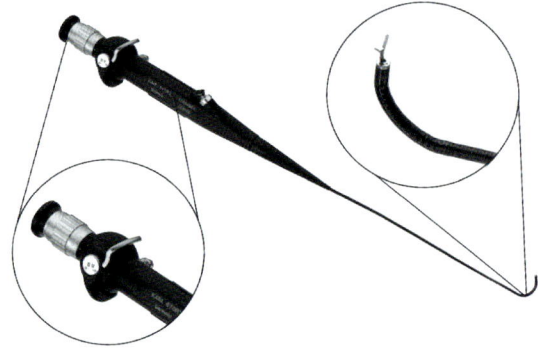

Fig 1.2: Karl Storz hystero-fibroscope

scopy the commonly used ones are of diameters (2 mm , 2.7 mm , 2.9 mm and 4 mm) with viewing angles 0°, 12.5° and 30°.

Telescopes are relatively fragile, and should be handled with special care avoiding any mechanical forces on them during operating , sterilizing and storing.

The hysteroscope is attached onto the telescope, with in turn is connected to a light source and a camera head (Fig. 1.4).

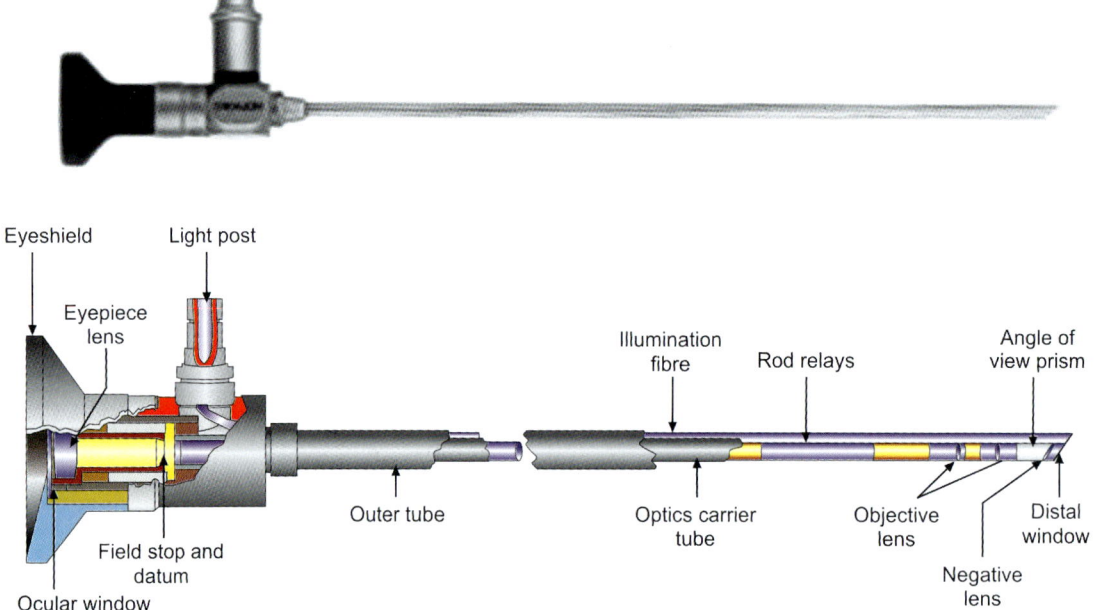

Fig 1.3: An endoscopic telescope

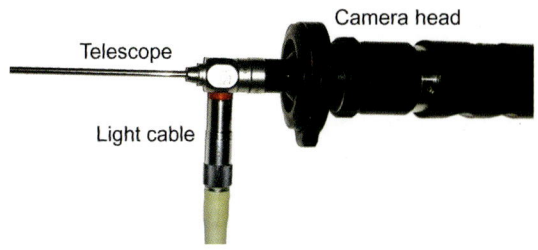

Fig. 1.4: Camera head and light cable attached to the telescope

Endoscopic Camera and Light Source

These are essential setup components in any endoscopic surgery. Hysteroscopy requires relatively basic camera and light source.

Light sources are devices with lamp inside (xenon, halogen or LED) and light is transferred to the telescope through an optic cable (Fig. 1.5).

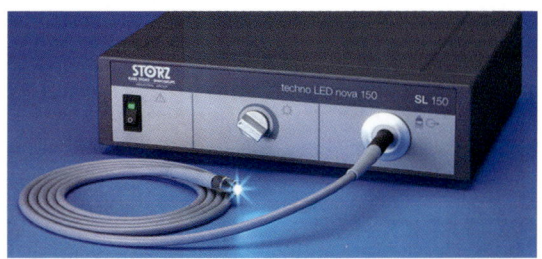

Fig. 1.5: LED light source with a light cable attached

The optic cable consists of hundreds of optic fibers, it is a fragile cable and susceptible to damage with direct impact, major twisting and crushing. It should not be stored, wind tighter than radius of 15 cm.

While operating with the light on, the distal end of the cable if unattached to the telescope, can cause burns.

Portable light sources are compact devices, with a battery and LED attached directly to the telescope, may be suitable for simple procedures (Fig. 1.6).

Cameras, as expected, have a very wide range of specifications, capabilities and costs. The higher the better, but more expensive. High-end cameras are not required to

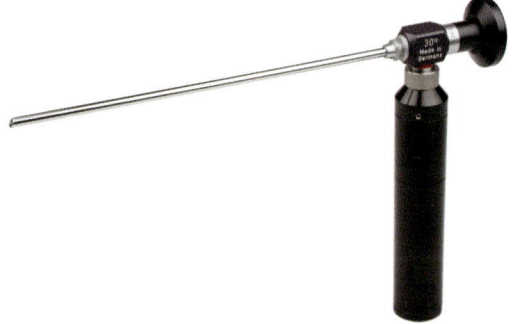

Fig. 1.6: A portable light source attached to a telescope

perform hysteroscopy.Three-chip cameras have better colors, HD cameras have better resolution, but all will work.

The camera head is attached to the telescope via a standard size coupling mechanism. Careful and gentle coupling of the telescope with camera head will avoid harming one of them (Fig. 1.7).

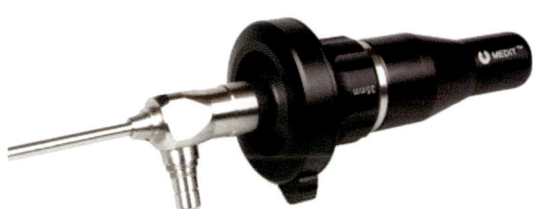

Fig. 1.7: Coupling of the telescope with camera head

Camera head will essentially have a "ring" to adjust the focus, and may have another ring for adjusting the zoom level.

The camera head is cable-connected to the camera control unit which processes the image and distributes it to a monitor or more, recording device or a network (Figs 1.8 and 1.9).

Image should be viewed on a suitable monitor, medical monitors are specialized for best image, but with higher costs. LCD monitors with resolution like or higher than the camera used will work fine.

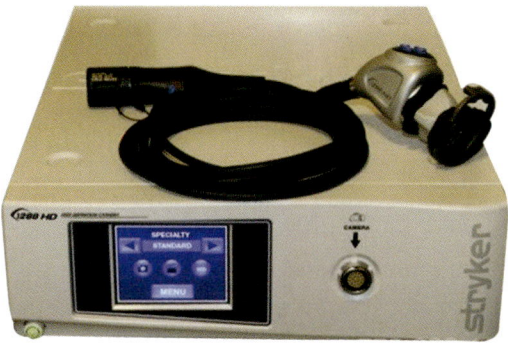

Fig. 1.8: Stryker HD camera system

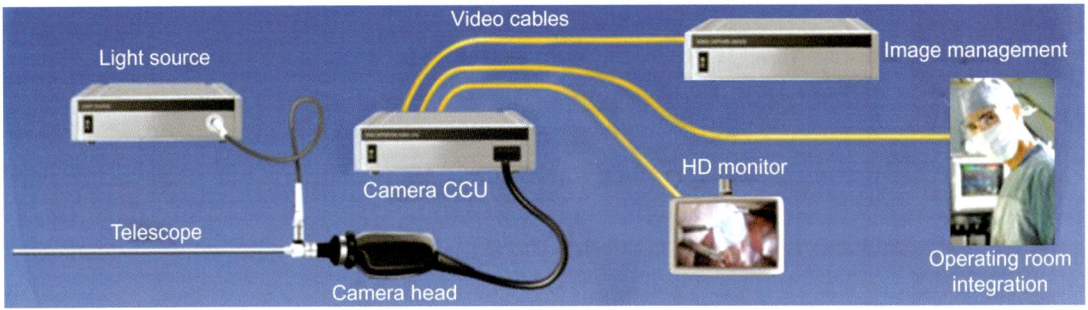

Fig. 1.9: Endoscopic visual setup

A video recording device is highly recommended for medical, legal and documentary issues. Specialized medical recorders are available, but again, all will work.

Endoscopic cameras have a "white balance" setting that calibrates the colors with the light before operating, a white gauze should be placed in front of the telescope, with light on, and the white balance button is pressed and focus adjusted.

Other modalities of the same devices are available, like the all-in-one devices, with a camera, light source, monitor and archiving system in one device (Fig. 1.10).

Electrosurgical Generator

Using electrosurgery in hysteroscopy is a common practice and an electric generator is required.

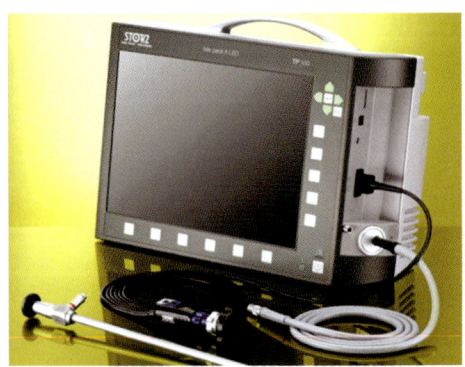

Fig. 1.10: Karl Storz Tele Pack X LED

Regular monopolar current can be used, but will require non-electrolytic distension media (distilled water or glycine) which are not as safe as saline. While regular bipolar current will not be powerful enough, there are special generators that provide "bipolar under saline" that are much safer, but again more expensive.

Distension Media Delivery Systems

Distension of the uterine cavity is mostly carried out by fluids, as carbon dioxide distension is not common any more due to its inconvenience.

Fluid distension is a very sensitive issue in hysteroscopic practice, as it is the most common cause of serious complications like fluid overload, air embolism and toxicity.

The amount of fluid used and intrauterine pressure are highly related to the technique of fluid delivery.

Automated pumps that measure the intrauterine pressure and keep it constant are optimal, but adds an extra cost on the setup as these can be substituted by techniques acquired from endourology like gravity-fed bags and pressure cuffs (Fig. 1.11).

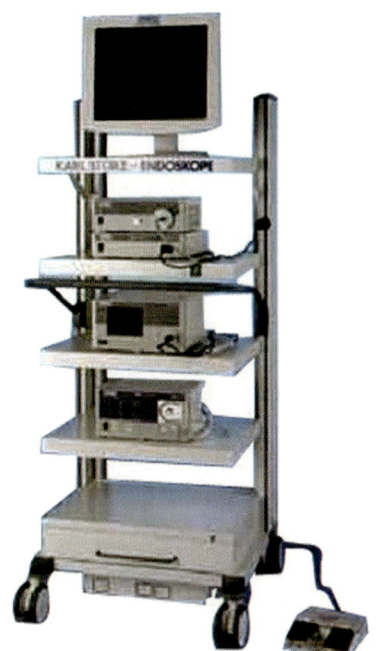

Fig. 1.12: An endoscopic tower

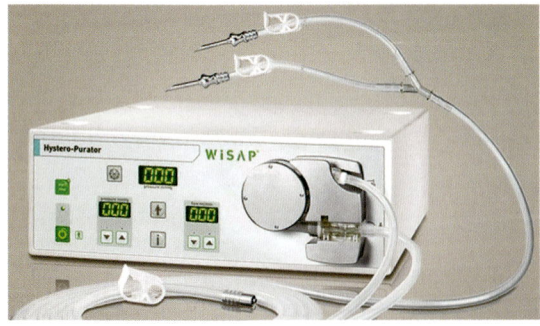

Fig. 1.11: Hystero-Purator automated hysteroscopy pump

All of the above equipment are put on an "endoscopic tower" (Fig. 1.12), with all connections and power supply (adding an UPS is also preferred to avoid electricity-related damage). The tower should have special care, minimal mobility and operated only by qualified personnel.

HYSTEROSCOPES AND INSTRUMENTS

Diagnostic Hysteroscope

It is simple, external sheath fixed around the telescope, with an inflow connection

allowing distension media to go into the cavity. Another design has an outflow connection to wash out the distension media. (Fig. 1.13).

The caliber of these hysteroscopes is slightly higher than the diameter of the telescope used (5 mm hysteroscope for the 4 mm telescope and 3.6 mm hysteroscope for the 2.9 mm telescope).

As the name defines, diagnostic hysteroscopes have no capabilities other than visualizing the inner cavity of the female genital tract, and any lesion will require the usage of another device.

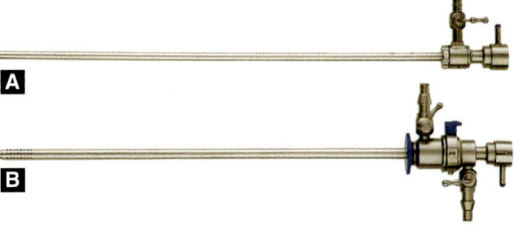

Fig. 1.13A and B: (A) Inflow-only diagnostic hysteroscope; (B) Below, continuous flow diagnostic hysteroscope

Operative Hysteroscopes

They are characterized by an additional "working channel" in which a variety of instruments can be inserted beside the telescope.

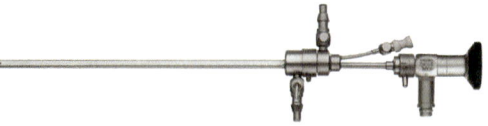

Fig. 1.14: Bettocchi office hysteroscope, size 5, by Karl Storz

The most famous design is the Bettocchi office hysteroscope, with an outer diameter of 5 mm, with a 2.9 mm 30° telescope and a 5 Fr wide working channel (which is also the inflow channel) (Fig. 1.14)

It consists of two sheaths (inner and outer) providing 4 openings (for telescope, inflow, outflow and a working channel). It is characterized by an oval profile rather than a circular one (Fig. 1.15)

There are countless other sizes and designs with same concept. A7 mm operative hysteroscope (with 4 mm telescope and 7 Fr working channel) and a 4 mm operative hysteroscope (with 2 mm telescope and 5 Fr working channel) are also available in market.

Campo Trophyscope from Karl Storz carries a new idea of sliding sheaths, can used as a diagnostic hysteroscope with 2.9 mm outer diameter (with a 2 mm telescope) then by sliding an operative sheath with a 5 Fr working channel, it becomes operative with a diameter of 4.4 mm (Fig. 1.16).

A recent modification of the office 5 mm hysteroscope is available from Tontarra, (modified inner sheath office hysteroscope)

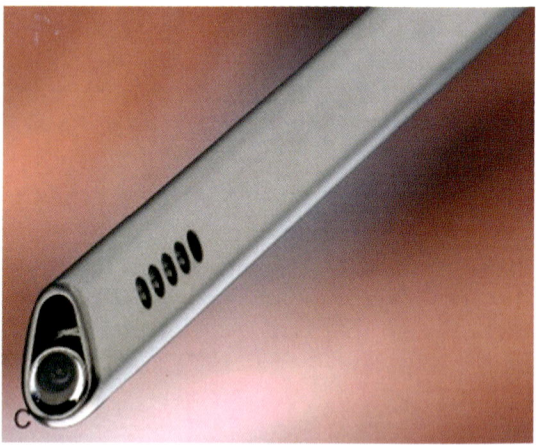

Fig. 1.15: Oval tip of Bettocchi hysteroscope

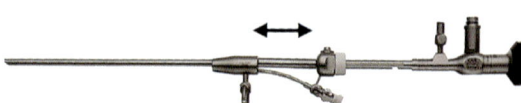

Fig. 1.16: Campo Trophyscope from Karl Storz

enables the usage of the internal sheath alone without the outer sheath, with a diameter of 4.4 mm and omitting the outflow for simple procedures (Fig. 1.17).

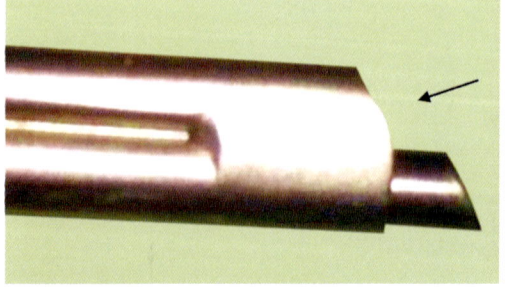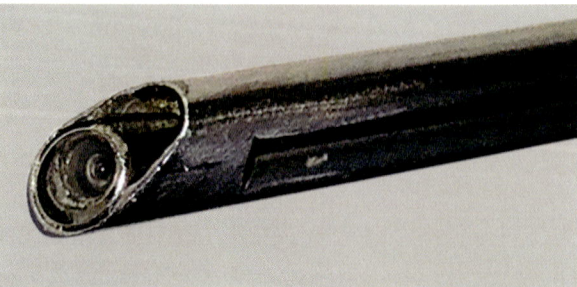

Fig. 1.17: Regular inner sheath (left) and a modified inner sheath office hysteroscope inner sheath tip (right)

Instruments used through the Working Channel

A variety of instruments can be utilized through the working channel into the uterine cavity to perform a wide range of different actions, they are categorized into as follows.

1. Mechanical Instruments

They resemble the laparoscopic instruments in form and function, different types of scissors and forceps are the most common and most important. Their main functions are to cut, grasp biopsy or foreign body (Fig. 1.18).

Other instruments with less common usage are also on the market, like palpation probe, myoma screw and hysterobasket.

Mechanical hysteroscopic instruments have a similar structure with a handle, shaft and working tip, the working tip and shaft has to have a caliber less than the working channel to allow their insertion (Fig. 1.19). They are malleable but not flexible, special care and training is required to handle and use them in the optimal way.

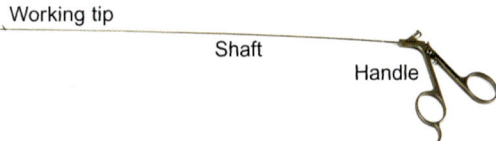

Fig. 1.19: 5 Fr hysteroscopic scissors

2. Hysteroscopic Electrodes

These are long isolated cylinders with electrode ends connected to either monopolar or bipolar circuit. They are handy and offer simple access to intrauterine electrosurgery, but in general, they are too small when it comes to big lesions and long operations.

Ball electrode, needle electrode, hook electrode are some examples (Fig. 1.20).

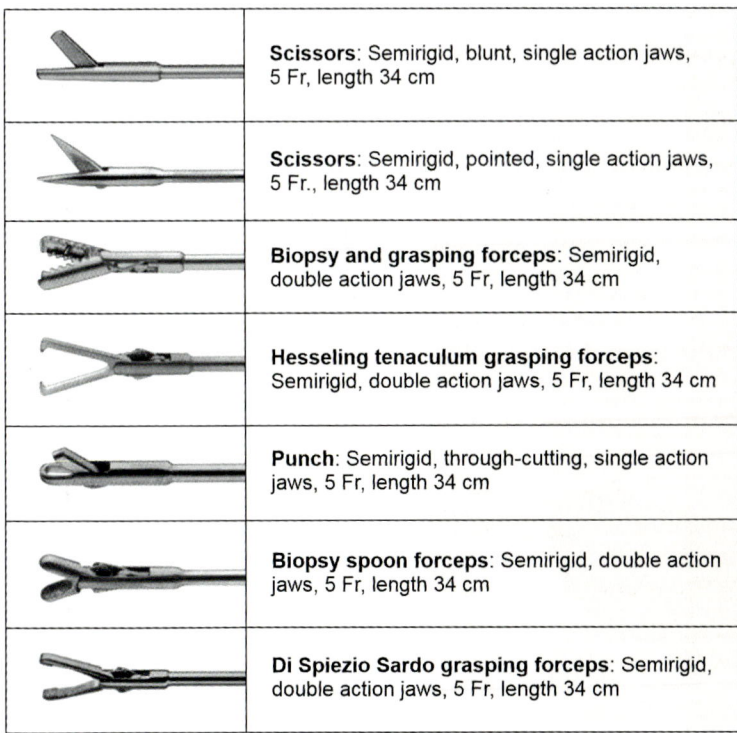

	Scissors: Semirigid, blunt, single action jaws, 5 Fr, length 34 cm
	Scissors: Semirigid, pointed, single action jaws, 5 Fr., length 34 cm
	Biopsy and grasping forceps: Semirigid, double action jaws, 5 Fr, length 34 cm
	Hesseling tenaculum grasping forceps: Semirigid, double action jaws, 5 Fr, length 34 cm
	Punch: Semirigid, through-cutting, single action jaws, 5 Fr, length 34 cm
	Biopsy spoon forceps: Semirigid, double action jaws, 5 Fr, length 34 cm
	Di Spiezio Sardo grasping forceps: Semirigid, double action jaws, 5 Fr, length 34 cm

Fig. 1.18: Different hysteroscopic scissors/forceps from Karl Storz

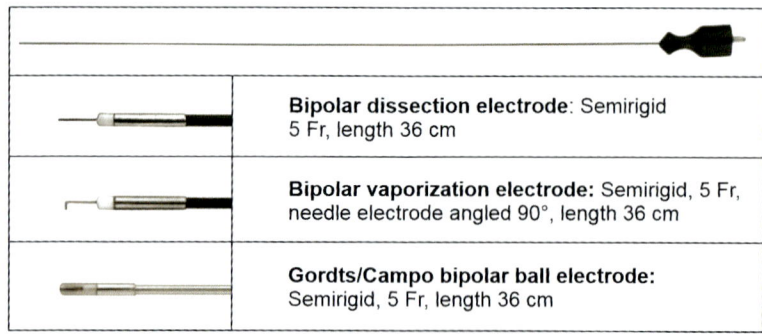

Bipolar dissection electrode: Semirigid 5 Fr, length 36 cm

Bipolar vaporization electrode: Semirigid, 5 Fr, needle electrode angled 90°, length 36 cm

Gordts/Campo bipolar ball electrode: Semirigid, 5 Fr, length 36 cm

Fig. 1.20: Bipolar 5 Fr hysteroscopic electrodes by Karl Storz

3. Laser Fibers

Intrauterine laser applications are not uncommon, as Nd-YAG and diode lasers have excellent cutting and coagulation effect, painless action, high safety profile and faster postoperative recovery times. Flexible laser fibers of suitable size are inserted through the working channel of operative hysteroscopes.

4. Other Special Tools

Fallopian tube cannulation set is a set of tubes with an inner hydrophobic rod inserted into the fallopian tube and traced using laparoscopy. It is inserted and, manipulated through an operative hysteroscope.

Many sterilization devices have utilized the operative hysteroscope as mode of application, like Essure and Ovibloc.

RESECTOSCOPES

Resectoscopes are a type of hysteroscopes that allow using relatively larger electrodes to operate. Electrodes are set on the resectoscopes form the front side ahead of the telescope, before inserting it into uterus rather than inserting it into a narrow working channel (Figs 1.21 and 1.22).

Resectoscopes are used for cutting, resection and ablation. They should only be used by experts, as the large electrodes and type of such operations carry more potential risk of complications.

The electrodes are fixed to a handle "working element" to control their movement back and forth, to avoid the over-travel away from field of view and their return back damaging the telescope. The default position of electrodes used in gynecology is being retracted, this is called "passive resectoscopes",

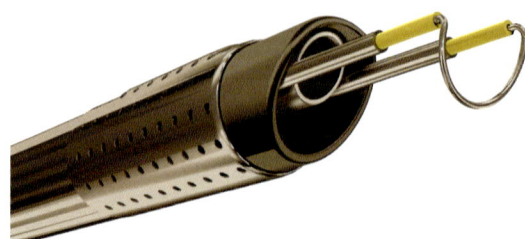

Fig. 1.21A: Tip of a resectoscope and a loop electrode in place

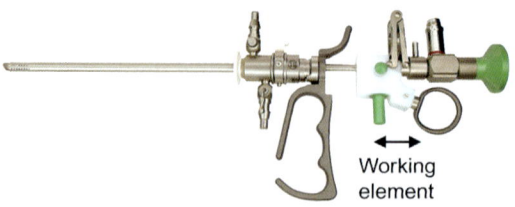

Working element

Fig. 1.21B: Monopolar resectoscope by Rudolf

on the other hand, urology surgeons prefer the "active resectoscopes" in which the electrodes default position is extended out.

There are many sizes of resectoscopes available, 26 Fr and 22 Fr were very common, newer devices with lower calibers are now in the market (16 Fr Gubbini hystero-resectoscope and 15 Fr mini resectoscope from Karl Storz) which can also be used in office.

Bipolar current is more safe and uses saline as distension media which is safer than monopolar current which needs a non-electrolytic solution like glycine. But because the bipolar electro-generator under saline is more expensive, many still use the mono-polar resectoscopes. Most recent resecto-scopes are hybrid, i.e. they can be used as both monopolar and bipolar devices.

Three main categories of electrodes are available with a wide variety of designs (Fig. 1.22)

- Loop electrodes for resection
- Knife electrodes for dissection
- Rollerball electrodes for ablation

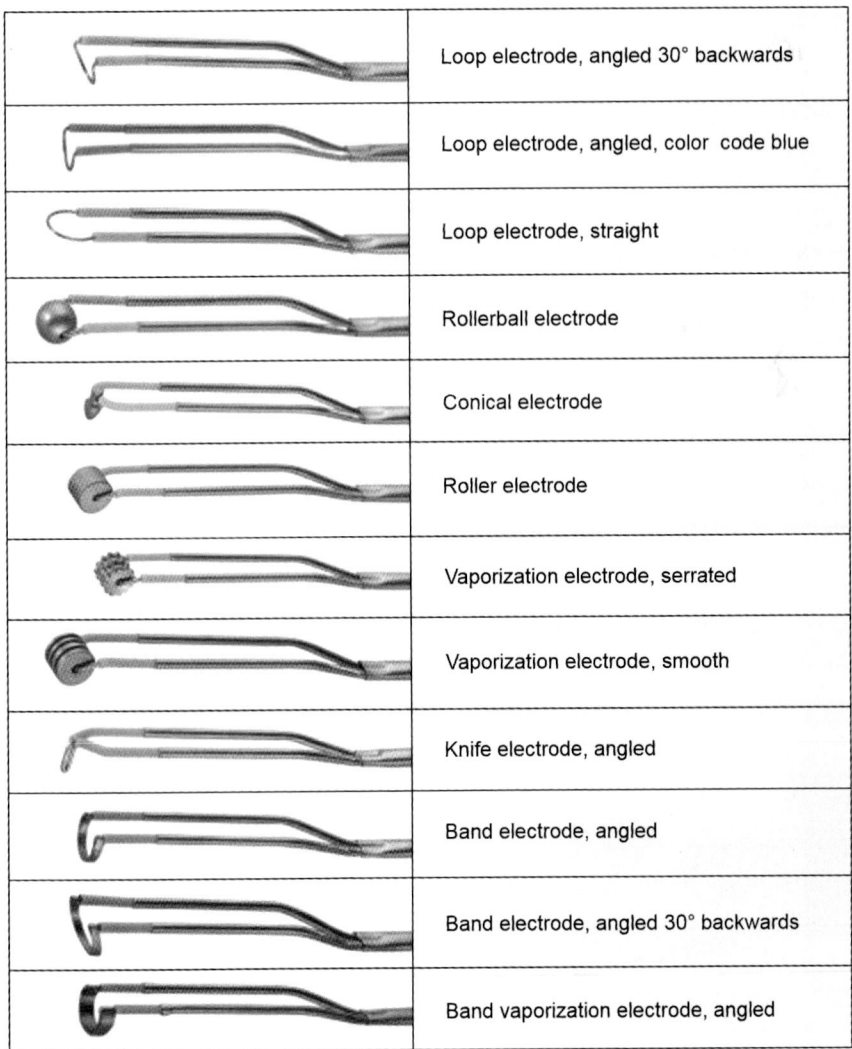

	Loop electrode, angled 30° backwards
	Loop electrode, angled, color code blue
	Loop electrode, straight
	Rollerball electrode
	Conical electrode
	Roller electrode
	Vaporization electrode, serrated
	Vaporization electrode, smooth
	Knife electrode, angled
	Band electrode, angled
	Band electrode, angled 30° backwards
	Band vaporization electrode, angled

Fig. 1.22: Some designs of resectoscope electrodes

Tissue Removal Systems

These are dedicated for operations that require extraction of a lesion from the intrauterine cavity (e.g. large polyps and fibroids), while resectoscopes resect the tissue and leave it in the cavity, blocking the vision and causing some inconvenience during operation, tissue removal systems resect and extract the tissue in the same time. They resemble the laparoscopic morcellator, with a continuous suction applied to the cutting end.

There are many known systems in the market like the MyoSure, Bigatti intrauterine shaver and TruClear (Fig. 1.23). Unfor-

tunately, they all use special telescopes and control units which add an additional cost on the setup.

Hystero-optics and Vaginoscopy

Using different angled telescopes in a tight space like the female genital tract is a bit tricky for beginners, as there would be a mismatching between "what is seen on the monitor" and "where the scope is directed".

Good understanding of how the angles telescopes work and how to deal with them will eliminate such a confusion and allow a smoother practice with less trauma to patient and instruments. In addition, this is the most

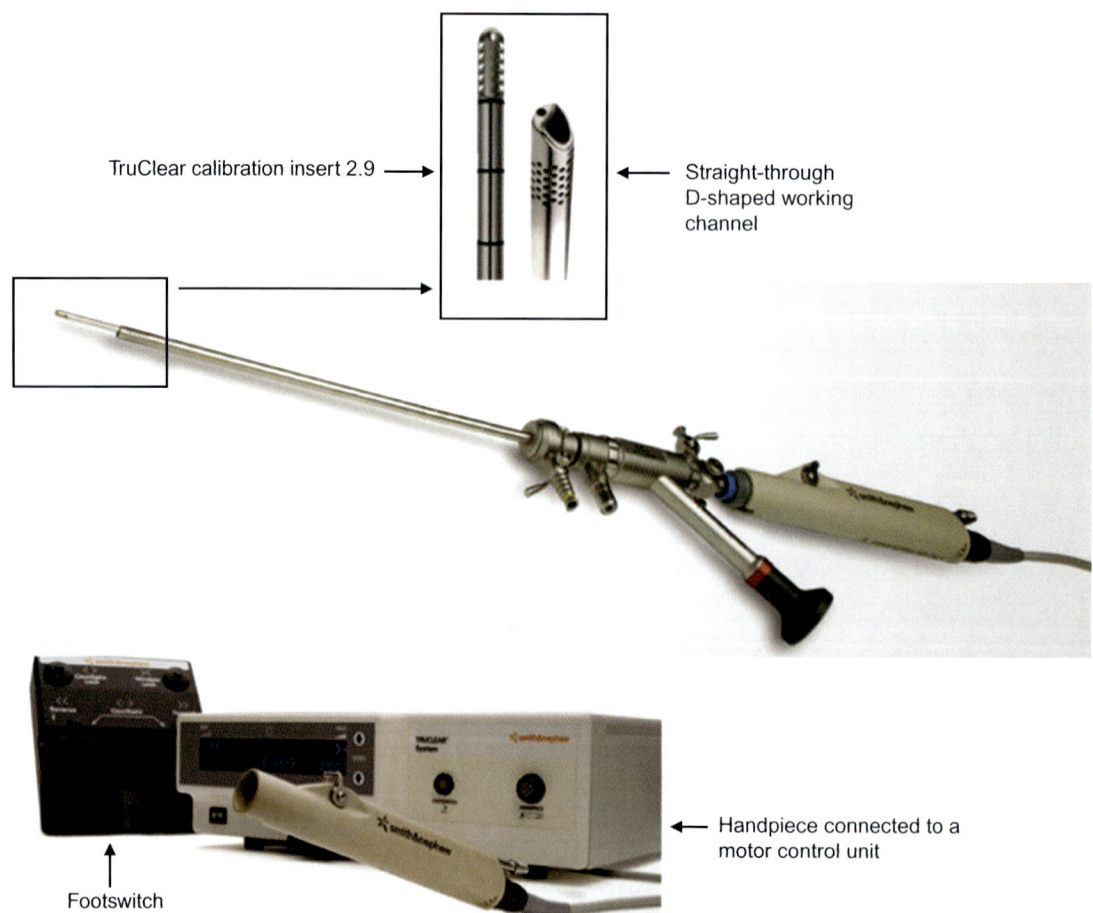

TruClear calibration insert 2.9 ⟶

Straight-through D-shaped working channel

Handpiece connected to a motor control unit

Footswitch

Fig. 1.23: TruClear system

important issue in vaginoscopic technique, the standard approach in office hysteroscopy.

In diagnostic and operative hysteroscopes, in addition to some resectoscopes, the telescopes used are 30° telescopes (Fig. 1.24). What does this mean?

The view on the beveled telescope is shifted to a direction by 30°. The view is still forward directed, but tilted to one side. This is called *foroblique view* (Fig. 1.24).

In Figure 1.25, the image on the monitor shows that point 1 is in front of the telescope, while this is untrue because the image is tilted upwards and the point in front of the axis of the telescope is point 2.

In other words, pushing the telescope forward, will make it go to point 2 not point 1. The angle between line 1 and line 2 is 30°.

Figure 1.26 shows the right view when inserting the telescope in a cylindrical narrow space (as the cervix) in the right direction, note the tunnel view and that the free area is in front of point 2 not point 1.

Figure 1.27 shows a trail to go into the cylinder by having its cavity centered, and as noted, the telescope is going into the lower wall of the cylinder.

Rotating the telescope around its axis will change the direction of the tilt (point 2 will rotate around point 1). There are two indicators by which the direction if tilting is known:

1. It is always opposite to the direction of light connector (tilted upward when the light connector is downward).
2. Most telescopes will have a "pointer" on the field of view to show the direction. The

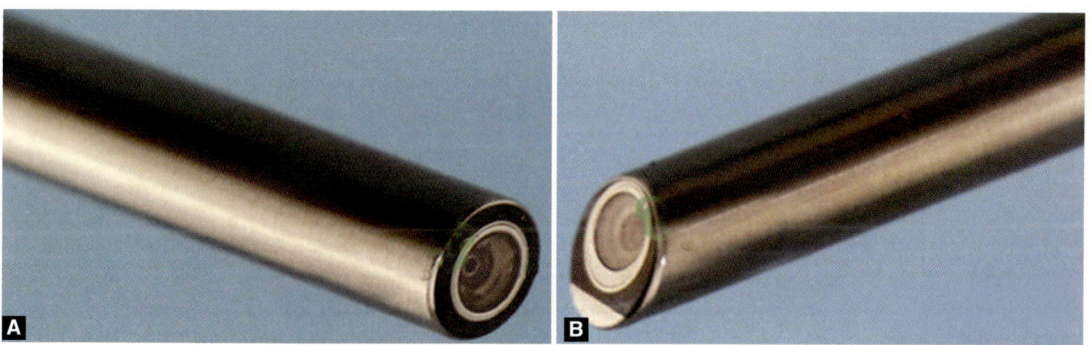

Fig. 1.24A and B: (A) 0° telescope; (B) 30° telescope

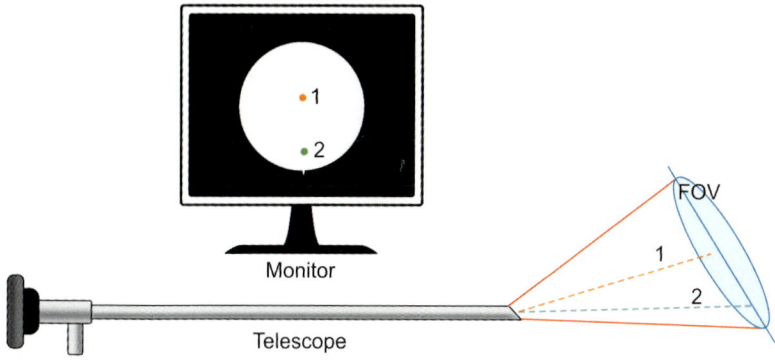

Fig. 1.25: Illustration of the foroblique view telescope. FOV: Field of view

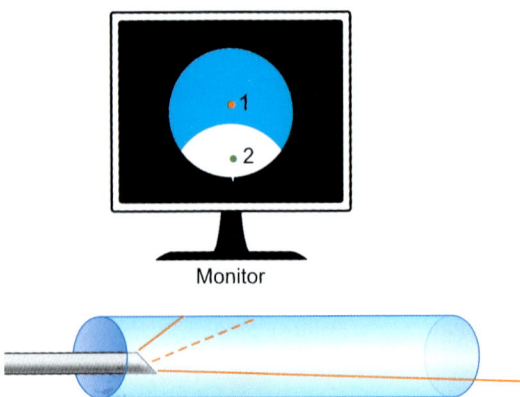

Fig. 1.26: Telescope in cylinder, right alignment

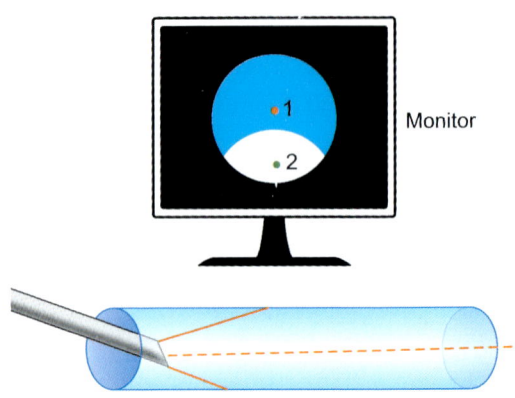

Fig. 1.27: Telescope in cylinder, wrong alignment

pointer is commonly placed in the direction of light connector (point 2) (Fig. 1.28) but sometimes, the pointer is on the other side.

Advantages of angled telescopes

- Wider field of view compared to 0° telescopes, as the view will change by rotating the telescope around its axis allowing vision in directions that cannot be accessed by 0° telescopes (Fig. 1.29A and B).
- Focused view for area of interest, this enables any point in the field of view to be brought to the center of view by rotating and manipulating the telescope, this allows better access to instruments to lesions in different places.

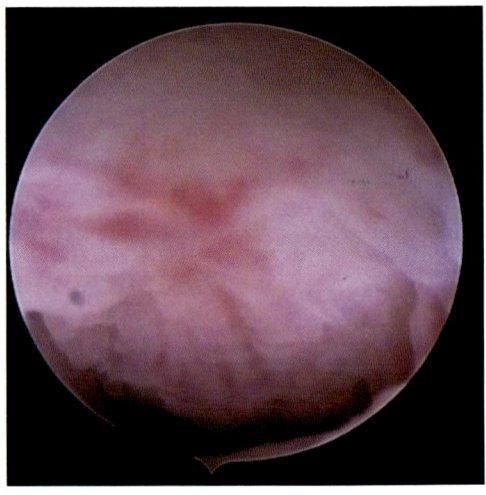

Fig. 1.28: Hysteroscopic view by a 30° telescope inside the cervix, the pointer is in the direction of the light connector, so point 2 is just above the pointer, note the tunnel-like view

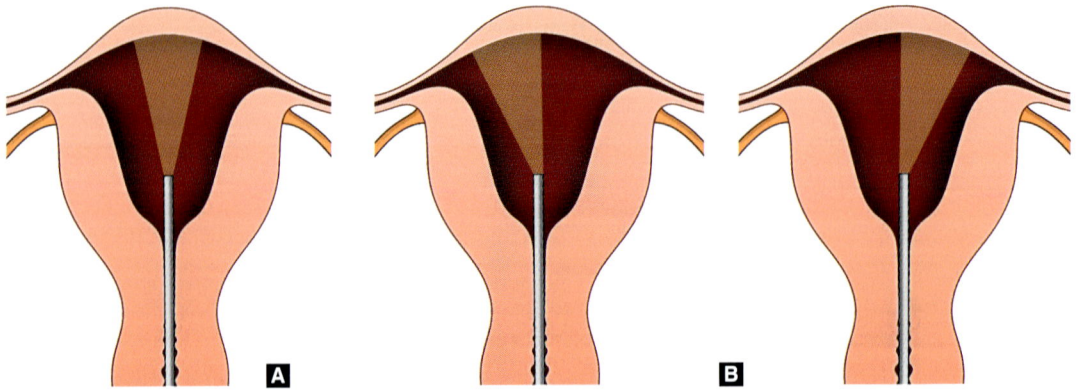

Fig. 1.29A and B: (A) 0° telescope; (B) 30° telescope manipulated by rotation

Vaginoscopic Approach

Vaginoscopy means accessing the uterine cavity by the hysteroscope without applying a vaginal speculum, cervical tenaculum or any other manual intervention. A non-touch technique based on manipulating the hysteroscope under vision through the vagina and cervix into the uterus.

This can only be done with hysteroscopes that have suitable calibers and will not need cervical dilatation. It is the standard technique in office hysteroscopy.

The fine skills of vaginoscopic approach depends on good understanding and clear imagination of the optical behavior of the angled telescopes along with knowing the female genital anatomy.

Detailed Steps of Vaginoscopy

Preparations

- Patient put in lithotomy position with perineum outside the bed lower edge.
- Patient covered and relaxed.
- Patient should see the monitor during the procedure.
- The hysteroscope attached to camera and light cable, light turned on.
- Make sure the camera is not mal-rotated. (view is upright on the monitor).
- Set white color and focus.
- Sit down on a swivel chair with wheels
- Connect the distension fluid tube to the inflow port.
- Open the valve to allow fluid to flow to eject air from the tubes and hysteroscope then close it.
- The hysteroscope is handled using the camera and rotated from the light connector of the telescope.
- Starting position is the light connector downward (telescope tilt is upward).

Procedure

1. Insert the hysteroscope into the vagina directing it posteriorly (in the direction on posterior fornix).
2. Allow the distension fluid to flow or turn on the distension pump, few seconds and the vagina will be filled. Closing the labia majora by hand from outside may help vaginal distension.
3. Inspect the vaginal walls and fornices.
4. Localize the cervix (hysteroscope directed downward and looking upward, the cervix should be see going into the posterior fornix) (Fig. 1.30).
5. Get nearer to the external os and avoid losing the view (Fig. 1.31).

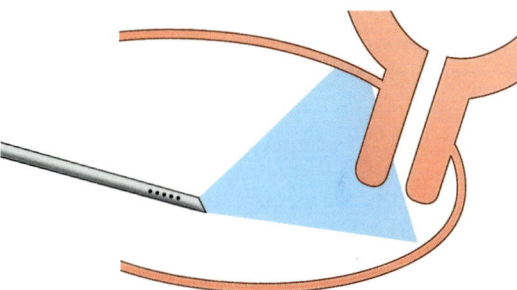

Fig. 1.30: Hysteroscope in vagina with cervix in field of view

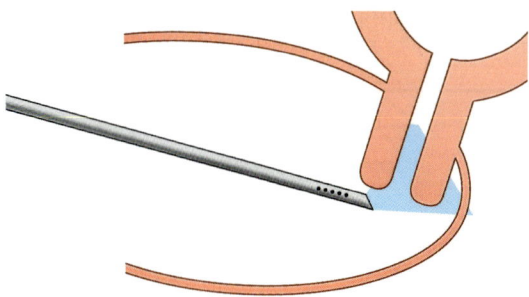

Fig. 1.31: Hysteroscope in vagina with cervix in center of field of view

6. Start entering the cervical canal, two things to consider:
   – The tunnel view, i.e. the posterior part of the os or canal should not be seen. (the os should be brought towards the pointer not towards the center of view).
   – The cervix is perpendicular to the vagina and in tilted upward, no wonder you may need the hysteroscope to have a vertical position. That is why the patient's perineum has to be outside the bed (Figs 1.32 and 1.33).

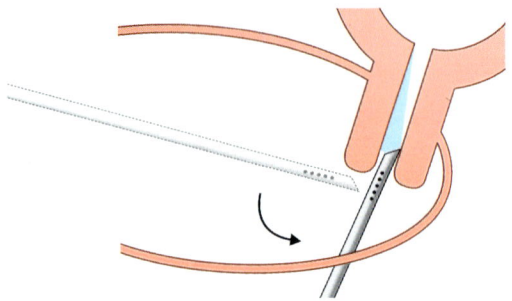

Fig. 1.32: hysteroscope changing direction and entering cervical canal

7. Travel into the cervical canal slowly, give time for hydrodistension and follow its direction.
8. At the internal os, it is recommended to rotate the hysteroscope 90° to alight the oval shape of the hysteroscope with the transverse oval shape of internal os, note the pointer rotates 90° too.
9. You should be inside the cavity now, rotate the hysteroscope back to its position.
10. There should be now an wide (panoramic) view of the cavity including the anterior wall.
11. Going few centimeters in towards the fundus then rotating the hysteroscope 90° towards left and right sides will show the lateral walls and ostia.

Using Instruments in Operative Hysteroscopy

As mentioned previously, mechanical instruments are delicate tools that need good

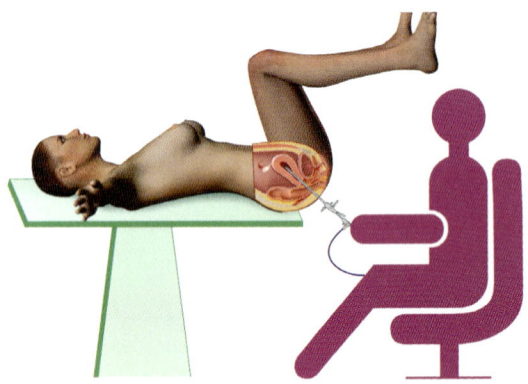

Fig. 1.33: Ideal patient and surgeon positioning. Note that the hysteroscope is directed upward

understanding, training and care during handling and usage.

Their insertion and passage through the working channel should be done carefully to avoid their damage, as the channel is relatively narrow and will not allow the instrument jaws to be opened inside it (Fig. 1.34).

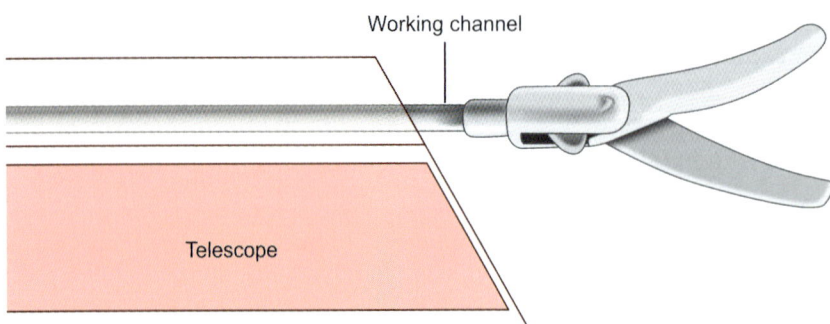

Working channel

Telescope

Fig. 1.34: Comparing the size of a 5 mm hysteroscope and its working channel to a 5 Fr opened scissors

The instrument should always be closed during insertion and extraction, and forceps should never be pulled outside while grasping anything.

The 30° tilting of view still causes some difficulty in interpreting the view with an instrument inserted. The working channel is in fixed position in relation to the telescope, in a way that the telescopic tilt is always "looking at" the instrument as soon as it leaves the channel (Fig. 1.34).

So once the instrument leaves the channel, it appears on one side of the view and travels to the other side on further insertion (Fig. 1.35). The optimal working site, is when the working tip is in the center of the view, further movement back or fro should be done using the hysteroscope itself with the instrument in it as one unit.

At the default position, the instrument will appear on the upper side of the view, work on anterior wall, anteroposterior adhesions and cutting into a septum is done in this position, but lateral and posterior wall lesions will need the hysteroscope to rotate to allow better view and easier access to the instrument to working area (Figs 1.36 and 1.37).

To conclude, familiarity with specifications, structure and functions of different tools is essential before performing any surgical intervention. Understanding the way things work, and good imagination of the optical process occurring is an important pillar for a good hysteroscopic operation. Keeping and handling the tools as per recommended, knowing how to sterilize every part in the right way, and using every instrument for its dedicated function are all parts of safe practice.

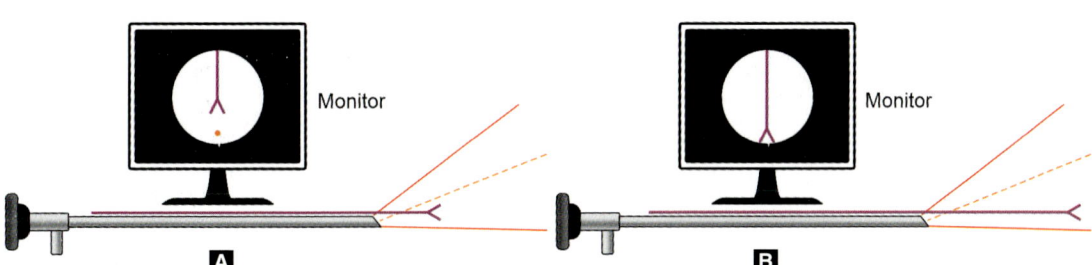

Fig. 1.35A and B: How inserting an instrument look like on the monitor

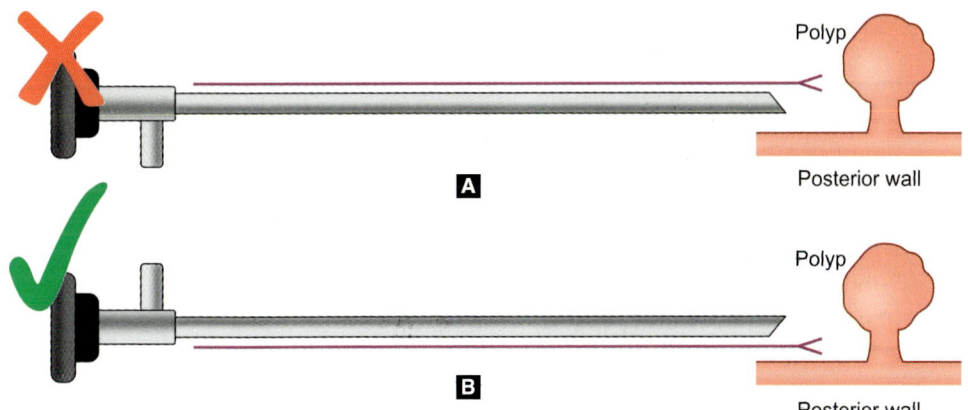

Fig. 1.36: Posterior wall polypectomy: (A) the wrong orientation and; (B) the right orientation

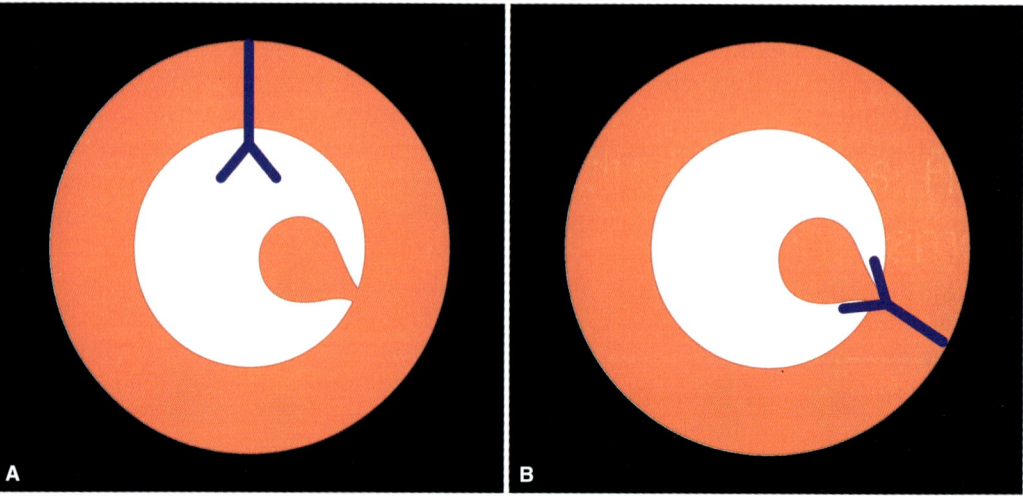

Fig. 1.37A and B: Rotating the hysteroscope to align with a polyp at 4 o' clock, note the position of the pointer and the instrument (in blue)

✍ Key Points

1. Hysteroscopy is not only clinical and surgical skills but also an appropriate knowledge of involved technologies and physical concepts is a must.
2. Tens of designs are available in the market for every tool, choose wisely.
3. Training is a fundamental part of good practice, enjoy it.
4. Instruments are delicate and fragile, take care.
5. Never miss the viewing angle; very useful, but tricky.
6. Office hysteroscopy = right tools + vaginoscopy.

BIBLIOGRAPHY

1. Andrea Tinelli, Luis Alonso Pacheco and Sergio Haimovich, Hysteroscopy, Springerlink, ISBN 978-3-319-57558–2, 2018
2. Hysteroscopes from KARL STORZ, Catalogue, www.karlstorz.com/cps/rde/xbcr/karlstorz_assets/ASSETS/3079310.pdf
3. "See Treat hysteroscopy in daily practice" PhD thesis by Attilio Di SpiezioSardo 2005- 2008. University of Naples, Faculty of Medicine http://www.fedoa.unina.it/3362/1/TESI_DOTTORATO_DI_SPIEZIO_SARDO.pdf
4. Sushma Deshmukh and Rahul Manchanda, Keynotes in Hysteroscopy, CBS Publishers, 2018

Uterine Distension Media: Types, Comparison and Recommendations

Fatema Ashraf, Rokeya Begum, Shahlagesmin

INTRODUCTION

Hysteroscopic diagnosis and surgical management can only be done properly, if uterine cavity is distended adequately. To allow a global view of the endometrial cavity, a befitting distension media, suitable for the activity, is obligatory. The ideal distending media should allow clear visualization of the uterine cavity, be isotonic, nontoxic, hypoallergenic, non-hemolytic, be rapidly cleared up by the body, readily available and inexpensive. However, which distension media suits best for diagnostic and operative hysteroscopy is still a matter of debate. Nevertheless, understanding the physical properties and the potential risks associated with the use of the various distending media is critical for the safe performance of hysteroscopic procedures .

Classification of the Distension Media

Distending media can be categorized as being either gaseous or fluid (Fig. 2.1). In regards to gaseous media, carbon dioxide is the only, to be used as distension media during hysteroscopy.

Fluid distending media can be classified according to viscosity, osmolality and presence or absence of electrolytes in the fluid (Table 2.1). Thus fluid media can be of

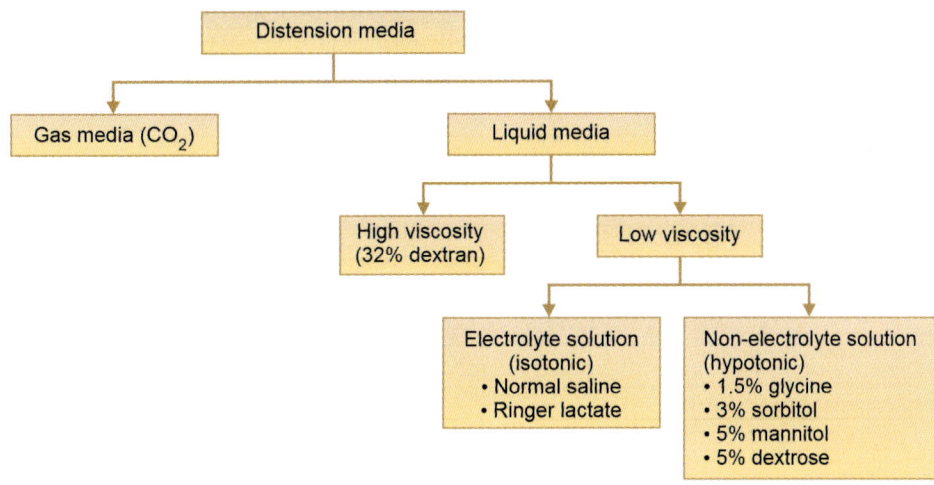

Fig. 2.1: Types of distension media

low or high viscosity, low or high molecular weight and can be either electrically conductive or nonconductive.

The high viscous solution used as distension media is dextran 32%. However, the low viscosity fluids can be divided into isotonic or hypotonic in relation to the osmolality of plasma (285 mOsm/L). Isotonic low viscosity fluids are 0.9% normal saline, Ringer's lactate solution and 5% mannitol. On the contrary, hypotonic low viscosity fluids are 1.5% Glycine, 3% sorbitol and 5% dextrose. Each medium has its own advantages and disadvantages, including specific safety concerns.

GASEOUS DISTENSION MEDIA

Carbon dioxide (CO₂)

Since 1972, Carbon dioxide gas, introduced by HJ. Lindemann (1920–2012), up to now is the only gaseous distension media used for hysteroscopy. In order to maintain an intracavitary pressure of 40–80 mmHg, an insufflation pressure of around 100–120 mmHg and a flow of 30–60 ml/min are needed, to distend the uterine cavity adequately with CO_2. It should be kept in mind that the safety threshold of pressure should be lower than 80–100 mmHg, that is essential to reduce the risk of embolism to a minimum. A dedicated electronic hystero-insufflator equipped with an automated system should be assigned for intrauterine pressure control (Fig. 2.2). Nowadays, carbon dioxide is used only in the field of diagnostic hysteroscopy.

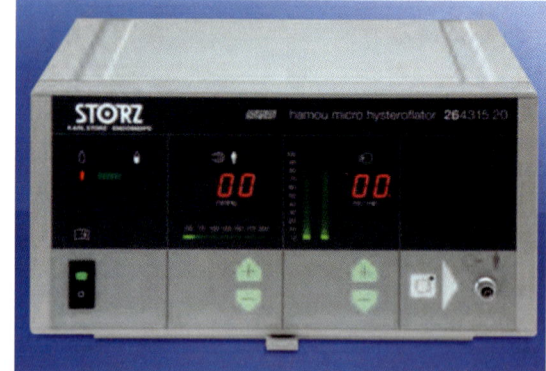

Fig. 2.2: Hamou Micro-Hysteroflator® SCB system for distension of uterine cavity by means of CO_2

Liquid Distension Media
1. High Molecular Weight High Viscosity Liquid Distension Media

The high viscosity high molecular weight medium used to distend the uterine cavity

Liquid media	Tonicity			Contains physiologic electrolytes			Viscosity	
	Iso	Hypo	Hyper	Yes	No	Low	High
Normal saline (NaCl .9%)	✓			✓		✓	
5% Glucose		✓			✓	✓	
1.5% Glycine		✓			✓	✓	
5% Dextrose (D5W)		✓			✓	✓	
5% Mannitol	✓				✓	✓	
3% Sorbitol		✓			✓	✓	
Mannitol/Sorbitol (Purisol)		✓			✓	✓	
32% Dextran 70 (Hyskon)			✓		✓		✓

Table 2.1: Characteristics of liquid distension media

is a solution of 32% dextran 70 in 10% glucose also known as Hyskon, which has the molecular weight of 70000 Daltons.

Administration

Commonly 100 ml is introduced into the uterus using the 50 ml syringe, sufficient to distend the uterine cavity adequately.

Advantages

Despite presence of blood, dextran 32% produces good visualization of the uterine cavity because of its low miscibility with blood, high light transmission capability and ease of use.

Disadvantages

The most important complications of Hyscon is intravascular expansion and cardiac failure. Because of its hyper osmolarity, small volumes absorbed can lead to disproportionate expansion of plasma volume. In a practical setting, 100 ml of solution administered intravenously can expand plasma volume by 870 ml resulting in vascular overload and subsequent heart failure and pulmonary edema. Furthermore, the use of dextran has been found to be associated with severe allergic reactions, hypersensitivity and case fatalities.

It is also worthy to know that, use of Hyskon tends to caramelize quickly on instruments, a feature that can lead to severe damage of the instruments. Because of its deadly complications at present it is no more used.

2. Liquid Low Molecular Weight and Low Viscous Distension Media

Low molecular weight distension media, unlike those with high molecular weight, require a continuous supply to permit an adequate and continuous intracavitary distension. These can be divided into non-electrolytes and electrolytes.

3. Liquid Low Molecular Weight Low Viscosity Non-electrolyte Distension Media

The electrolyte-free lowviscosity media include 3% sorbitol, 1.5% glycine, 5% mannitol, and combined solutions of sorbitol and mannitol. The typical combination is a mixture of 3% sorbitol and 0.5% mannitol. The non-electrolyte solutions (glycine, sorbitol and mannitol) having neither cations nor anions, are incapable to conduct electricity, thus they can be safely employed in hysteroscopy, while using unipolar electrosurgical systems.

Sorbitol

Sorbitol is a reduced form of dextrose (D-glucitol) and an isomer of mannitol. When absorbed systemically they are either excreted intact by the kidney or rapidly metabolized by the fructose pathway to CO_2 and water.

Glycine

Glycine is a nonconductive amino acid with a plasma half-life of 85 minutes. The component is uniquely metabolized in the liver producing ammonia and free water, which can result in further reductions of serum osmolality.

Mannitol

Mannitol (D-mannitol), a 6-carbon polyol that occurs in nature, is often called a sugar alcohol, and is an isomer of sorbitol. Solutions of mannitol are isotonic when mixed with water at a concentration of 5%, and because it is not absorbed by the renal tubules, it functions as an osmotic diuretic by increasing both sodium and extracellular water excretion.

4. Liquid Low Molecular Weight Low Viscosity Electrolyte Distension Media

Normal saline (NS)

Normal saline (NS) and other isotonic electrolyte-rich solutions are useful and safer media. Normal saline is a good choice for minor office procedures and the use of saline solution is imperative when using bipolar electrodes.

Ringer's Lactate

Ringer's lactate possesses similar properties as normal saline but more physiological and consequently would be expected to have a similar risk profile. However, no studies were identified that specifically evaluated the use of Ringer's lactate for hysteroscopic applications on account of its infrequent use as a medium for hysteroscopy.

Advantages of Liquid Low Molecular Weight Distension Media

On the order of allowing good endoscopic vision each of the low molecular weight solutions provides excellent visibility for the endoscopic surgeries. Uterine distension using saline solution is associated with an increased level of patient compliance. However, even if there is absorption of a substantial volume, normal saline does not cause electrolyte imbalance. A better cost-benefit ratio in cases of intrauterine bleeding, compared to those modalities using carbon dioxide emphasize its demand in the field of hysteroscopic surgery.

Disadvantages of Liquid Low Molecular Weight Distension Media

Normal saline is associated with fewer unfavorable changes in serum sodium and osmolality than is the case when electrolyte-free media are used with monopolar systems. Absorption of an excessive amount of the irrigation fluid may rarely lead to fluid overload and causes operative hysteroscopy intravascular absorption (OHIA) syndrome. However, use of glycine, has the potential risk of neurotoxicity.

Administration of Liquid Distension Media

A liquid distension medium can be administered:

- At atmospheric pressure: Two bags 3 or 5 liters are connected through a urological 'Y' tubing set (Fig. 2.3) and positioned 90–100 cm from the patient's perineal plane, in order to generate an irrigation pressure of about 70 mmHg.
- By means of pressure generated by an instrument similar to a blood pressure monitor, the 'squeeze-bulb' (80–120 mmHg) is used (Fig. 2.4).

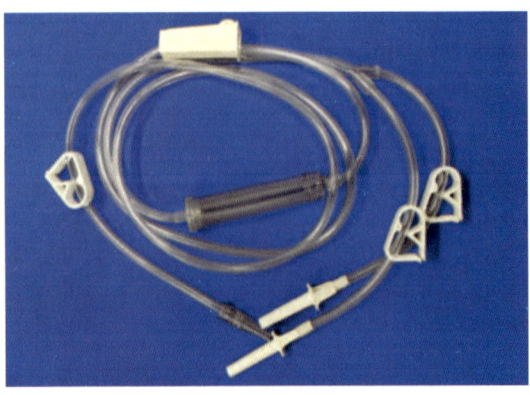

Fig. 2.3: "y" tubing set

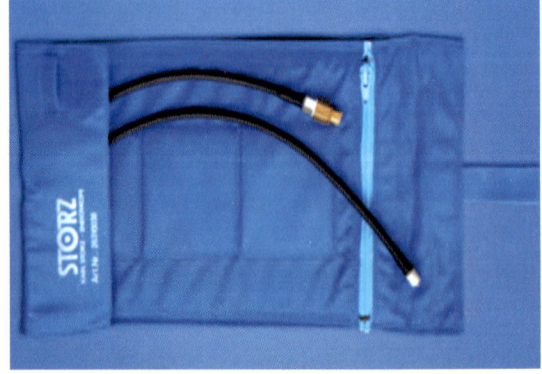

Fig. 2.4: Squeeze bulb

- Wherefore an automated microprocessor-controlled irrigation and suction unit can be employed to enable a clear field of vision and maintains a constant and optimal level of uterine distension.

Precautions for Different Distension Media

Uterine distension pressures need to be sufficient to allow systematic inspection of the entire uterine cavity. However, care is needed to ensure that pressures are minimized to avoid over distension of the uterus and consequent pain.

Precaution for CO_2

CO_2 should be delivered to the endometrial cavity through the sheath of the hystero-scopic system from an insufflator designed specifically for hysteroscopy, which regulates pressure and gas flow. The insufflator can be a separate unit or a small cartridge attached via a handle of the hysteroscopic system. It is essential that a low-pressure hysteroscopic insufflator be used and not a laparoscopic or other type of endoscopic insufflator, which typically inflate with much higher pressures. The use of such instruments for hysteroscopy could be associated CO_2 embolism which can be fatal for the patient.

Precaution for Liquid Media

Particular care is required with resection of the endometrium (transcervical resection of the endometrium TCRE) and hysteroscopic myomectomy (transcervical resection of fibroids—TCRF), where a large amount of fluid is introduced and vessels remain opened up. Precaution must be taken during use of large diameter endoscopes with high rates of media inflow especially in procedures that involve FIGO type I/II fibroids, metroplasty and endometrial resection. To minimize the risk of air embolism, the hysteroscope and inflow

tubing should be primed with the fluid media to eliminate air bubbles before inserting the hysteroscope into the uterine cavity. Consequently, after using hyskon or similar solutions instruments should be thoroughly cleaned with warm water after every procedure. Admittedly, when used, the clinician must be prepared for the rare case of anaphylaxis, and should practice detailed and strict protocols.

Complications Imposed by Distension Media

During operative hysteroscopy absorption of large volumes of distension solutions can occur leading to serious complications arising from significant fluid overload. Excessive fluid absorption is most likely with prolonged hysteroscopic procedures requiring continuous irrigation of fluid or where blood vessels within the myometrium are opened.

Complications in using High Viscous Media

The major problems related to dextran 70 are plasma volume expansion, threatening life and anaphylaxis.

Complications related to hypotonic, non-electrolyte fluid media

Glycine 1.5 % (200 mOsm/L) and sorbitol 3% (165 mOsm/L) use if crosses the normal threshold of absorption causes hyper-volemia and consequent dilutional hypona-tremia. Symptoms usually develop when serum sodium concentration drops below 125 mmol/L.

Sorbitol 3% is a hypotonic sugar solution and if excessive intravasation of sorbitol occurs, it can also lead to hyperglycemia and hypocalcemia. Consequent symptoms can develop quite rapidly, including myoclonus within an hour of the procedure has been described.

Complications Related to Isotonic Electrolyte Fluid Media

Although isotonic electrolyte fluid media is comparatively safe, but if absorbed in large amount, has the potential to cause congestive cardiac failure and pulmonary edema.

Complications Related to Gaseous Media

CO_2 is highly soluble in blood, therefore, if large volumes of CO_2 reaches the systemic circulation, life threatening cardiorespiratory collapse may occur. Air or gas embolism is rare but can occur during a hysteroscopy with both gas (CO_2) or fluid distension media.

Risk of Air Embolism

Air can enter the uterine cavity during insertion of the hysteroscope if the inflow tubing is not primed with fluid or due to air bubbles within the distension medium potentially causing air embolism. Gas embolism may arise from the combustion and gases produced during hysteroscopic electrosurgery.

Clinically significant gas embolism is considered to be quite rare and there are relatively few case reports published in the literature.

Choosing a Distension Media

When selecting distention media for hysteroscopy, a number of factors should be considered including the procedure to be performed and the instruments to be used, particularly those that require radio frequency and electricity.

If monopolar electrosurgical instruments are to be used, the distending medium should not contain electrolytes, as energy would get dissipated during the surgical procedure; hence electrolyte free solutions have to be used with monopolar energy.

In contrary, if mechanical or bipolar electrosurgical instruments are to be used, then normal saline is the better choice because of better patient compliance and its cost effectiveness.

During office hysteroscopy, there are no significant difference in perceived pain between carbon dioxide and normal saline medium.

Findings suggest that the advantages of CO_2 are limited, but do not preclude its use in selected clinical situations when appropriately used.

CHOICE BETWEEN FLUID AND GASEOUS MEDIA

Carbon dioxide is used for diagnostic hysteroscopy, as bleeding during operative procedures obscures visibility. Presence of blood and debris and the risk of gas embolism render CO_2 unsuitable to use in operative hysteroscopy. Fluid media are most suitable when undertaking operative procedures. The advantage of fluid over CO_2 gas is the symmetric distension of the uterus with fluid and its effective ability to flush blood, mucus, bubbles, and small tissue fragments out of the visual field.

Choice within the fluid media

Amongst the fluid media, the choices are between an isotonic or hypotonic fluid depending upon the energy modality used. Isotonic fluids may contain electrolytes such as sodium chloride and Ringer's lactate solution or are electrolyte free such as mannitol, although the latter is rarely used. Electrolyte solutions are used with bipolar energy and with mechanical procedures such as morcellation of submucosal fibroids and endometrial polyps. Electrolyte containing fluids are not be effective when using monopolar energy.

Fluid Deficit Monitoring

Fluid deficit, also known as the fluid, absorbed into the systemic circulation is an important concern during hysteroscopy. Accurate measurement of the amount of the introduced and absorbed media at all times, is always a must.

But accurate calculation is practically difficult and complicated by following factors:

1. It might be difficult to collect all the media that passes out of the uterus during the procedure and that falls on the floor of the operating room.
2. The actual volume of media solution in 3 L bags is typically more than the labelled volume.
3. Difficulties in estimating the volume of media left in a used or "emptied" infusion bag.
4. Systemic absorption that in some instances may occur extremely rapidly.

The simplest method of monitoring comprises manually subtracting the volume collected from the volume infused considering all sources including the hysteroscope or resectoscope outflow; the 'perineal' collection drape, which includes a pouch to capture fluid spilled from the cervix but around the hysteroscope sheath; and the media spilled that is collected on the floor. However, while conceptually simple, there are a number of difficulties encountered when attempting to collect media from all sources in the operating room environment.

The limitations of manual measurement make it preferable to use an automated fluid measurement system that takes into account an exact measurement of infused volume as well as all of the potential sources of returned media. Such systems provide continuous measurement of the amount of distending media absorbed into the systemic circulation by using the weight of the infused volume.

BSGE/ESGE 2018 Defines Fluid Overload

- *Hypotonic* solution overload-fluid deficit threshold of **1000 ml** in healthy women of reproductive age and **750 ml** for elderly women or with cardiac and renal co-morbidities.
- *Isotonic* solution overload-fluid deficit threshold of **2500 ml** in healthy women of reproductive age and **1500 ml** for elderly women or with cardiac and renal co-morbidities.

Fluid deficit of 1000 ml has traditionally been the threshold when using hypotonic media, at which point the procedure should be curtailed in women of reproductive age. While using 1.5% glycine, a decrease of 10 mmol/L in serum sodium level indicates absorption of approximately 1000 ml distension media.

BSGE/ESGE 2018 Executive Committee: Safety Recommendations

- Isotonic, electrolyte-containing distension media such as normal saline should be used with mechanical instrumentation and bipolar electrosurgery because of low risk of hyponatraemia and fluid overload
- Hypotonic, electrolyte-free distension media such as glycine and sorbitol should only be used with monopolar electro-surgical instruments.
- Carbon dioxide gaseous media should be used for diagnostic hysteroscopy only.
- Automated pressure delivery systems provides constant intrauterine pressure and accurate fluid deficit surveillance, advantageous in prolonged operative procedures.
- Measurement of the fluid deficit should be done at a minimum of 10 min intervals
- Local anesthesia with sedation should be considered for performing operative hysteroscopic procedures rather than general anesthesia.

✍ Key Points

1. The simplest diagnostic—only hysteroscopic procedures utilize a fluid or gaseous uterine distending media while fluid media is the only choice for operative hysteroscopy, to allow clear and adequate view.
2. The fluid media is further classified into electrolyte-poor and electrolyte-rich categories. These two media are used with monopolar and bipolar electrical systems respectively.
3. Excessive absorption of any fluid media can lead to fluid overload. The most alarming complication is intravasation of large volumes of electrolyte-poor media which may result in hyponatremia.
4. For hysteroscopy using a fluid distending medium, an automated rather than a manual fluid monitoring system should be adopted.
5. Regarding hysteroscopy using an electrolyte fluid media, procedure should be halted at a fluid deficit of 2500 mL in otherwise healthy women below 50 years. For others, the threshold has to be individualized according to cardiovascular status.
6. Use of carbon dioxide for uterine distension requires insufflation with a hysteroscopic insufflator. A laparoscopic insufflator should never be used because of its potential of causing gas embolism.
7. Air embolism is a rare complication of hysteroscopy. It may occur when carbon dioxide is used as a medium or, if air bubbles are introduced while using fluid media. Dyspnea is the most common symptom.
8. If any complication is suspected, the procedure must be terminated immediately, the uterus should be deflated, sources of fluid or gas removed, and supportive care should be ensured.

BIBLIOGRAPHY

1. Almonti S, Cipriani AM, Villani V, Rinalduzzi S. Reversible myoclonus in a patient undergoing transcervical hysteroscopic surgery. Neurological sciences: official journal of the Italian Neurological Society and of the Italian Society of Clinical Neurophysiology 2013;34(10):1815–7.
2. Brandner P, Neis KJ, Ehmer C. The etiology, frequency, and prevention of gas embolism during CO_2 hysteroscopy. The Journal of the American Association of Gynecologic Laparoscopists. 1999;6(4):421–8.
3. Brooks PG. Venous air embolism during operative hysteroscopy. The Journal of the American Association of Gynecologic Laparo-scopists. 1997;4(3):399–402.
4. Brusco GF, Arena S, Angelini A. Use of carbon dioxide versus normal saline for diagnostic hysteroscopy. Fertility and sterility. 2003;79(4): 993–7.
5. Darwish AM, Hassan ZZ, Attia AM, Abdelraheem SS, Ahmed YM. Biological effects of distension media in bipolar versus monopolar resectoscopic myomectomy: a randomized trial. Journal of Obstetrics and Gynaecology Research. 2010;36(4):810–7.
6. Di Spiezio Sardo A, Minozzi S, Gubbini G, Casadio P. Practical guideline in office hysteroscopy. 2011–2012.
7. Hawe JA, Chien PF, Martin D, Graham Phillips A, Garry R. The validity of continuous automated fluid monitoring during endometrial surgery: luxury or necessity? BJOG: An International Journal of Obstetrics and Gynaecology. 1998;105(7):797–801.
8. Imasogie N, Crago R, Leyland NA, Chung F. Probable gas embolism during operative hysteroscopy caused by products of combustion. Canadian Journal of Anesthesia. 2002;49 (10):1044–7.
9. Istre O, Bjoennes J, Naess R, Hornbaek K, Forman A. Postoperative cerebral oedema after transcervical endometrial resection and uterine irrigation with 1.5% glycine. Lancet. 1994; 344(8931):1187–9.
10. Mangar D. Anaesthetic implications of 32% Dextran-70 (Hyskon) during hysteroscopy: hysteroscopy syndrome. Canadian journal of anaesthesia = Journal canadien d'anesthesie. 1992;39(9):975–9.
11. Mencaglia L, Lugo E, Consigli S, Barbosa C. Bipolar resectoscope: the future perspective of hysteroscopic surgery. Gynecological surgery. 2009;6(1):15.
12. Munro MG, Critchley HO, Broder MS, Fraser IS. FIGO classification system (PALM-COEIN) for causes of abnormal uterine bleeding in nongravid women of reproductive age. International journal of gynaecology and obstetrics: the official organ of the International Federation of Gynaecology and Obstetrics. 2011;113(1):3–13.

13. Munro MG, Storz K, Abbott JA, Falcone T, Jacobs VR, Muzii L, et al. AAGL Practice Report: Practice Guidelines for the Management of Hysteroscopic Distending Media: (Replaces Hysteroscopic Fluid Monitoring Guidelines. J Am Assoc Gynecol Laparosc. 2000;7:167–168.). Journal of minimally invasive gynecology. 2013;20(2):137–48.

14. Nappi C, Sardo ADS. State-of-the-art Hysteroscopic Approaches to Pathologies of the Genital Tract: Endo-Press; 2014.

15. Touboul C, Fernandez H, Deffieux X, Berry R, Frydman R, Gervaise A. Uterine synechiae after bipolar hysteroscopic resection of submucosal myomas in patients with infertility. Fertility and sterility. 2009;92(5):1690–3.

16. Umranikar S, Clark TJ, Saridogan E, Miligkos D, Arambage K, Torbe E, et al. BSGE/ESGE guideline on management of fluid distension media in operative hysteroscopy. Gynecological surgery. 2016;13(4):289–303.

17. Witz CA, Silverberg KM, Burns WN, Schenken RS, Olive DL. Complications associated with the absorption of hysteroscopic fluid media. Fertility and sterility. 1993;60(5):745–56.

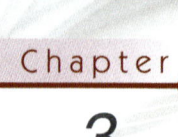

Techniques: Diagnostic and Operative Office Hysteroscopy

Richa Sharma, Rahul Manchanda

Office hysteroscopy (OH) or outpatient hysteroscopy (OPH)

Diagnostic and operative hysteroscopy are done in the office or outpatient settings outside the formal operation theater.

In modern era, office hysteroscopy can be considered as the gold standard for the examination of the uterine cavity and overcoming the significant limitations of D and C and other blind techniques. However, the success of office hysteroscopy, either diagnostic or operative depends upon several tips and tricks (Flowchart 3.1).

Flowchart 3.1: Office hysteroscopy

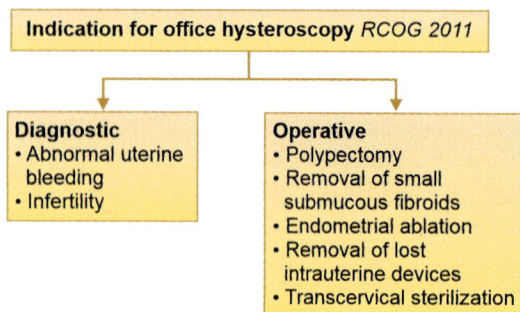

Success of Office Hysteroscopy

It depends upon following components

1. Comfortable setting
2. Favorable anatomical characteristics of the uterus
3. Miniaturization of equipment

4. Vaginoscopy
5. Saline solution as a distension medium
6. Expertise—specific hysteroscopic training

1. Comfortable Setting (Fig. 3.1)

Outpatient hysteroscopy should not be performed in a formal operating theatre.

- It should be a dedicated hysteroscopy suite or a multipurpose facility room of appropriately sized and fully equipped treatment room.
- Private and patient friendly, with a separate, and adjoining, changing area with a toilet facilities that minimizes her anxiety.
- Adequate resuscitation facilities, comfortable recovery area with refreshment-making facilities
- At least **3 support staff** consisting of at least 1 registered general nurse and healthcare assistants, one for **'Vocal Local'** Communication with the woman for reassurance, explanation and support, helps to alleviate anxiety and divert their attention, thus minimising pain and embarrassment.
- Surgeon should involve the patient by inviting her to look at the additional monitors and explain the views or any other abnormalities found, this drastically minimizes the anxiety and pain.

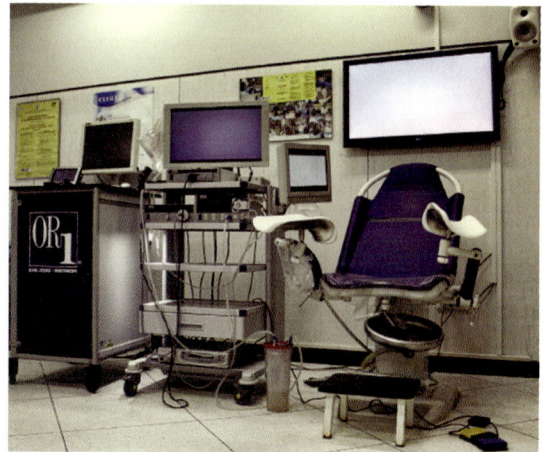

Fig. 3.1: Comfortable setting

- Simple written patient information leaflet should be provided, along with clear informed choices (see or see and treat' services)
- Accordingly formal consent be taken before the procedure, including for analgesics and anesthetics.

2. Favorable Anatomical Characteristics of the Uterus

Sensitive innervations of the uterus are present at myometrium, serosal surface and only basal thirds of endometrium. Also any fibrotic tissue or lesions within the cavity are not pain sensitive, thus the procedures at superficial endometrium can be carried out

without analgesia or anesthesia, e.g. polypectomy, submucous myomectomy G0,1 and flimsy adhesiolysis (Fig. 3.2A to C).

3. Miniaturization of equipment

The cervical canal is typically 3–4 cm in length and 3 cm in diameter. The narrowest location of the cervical canal is by nature extendable to a diameter of 5 mm, without pain (Fig. 3.3)

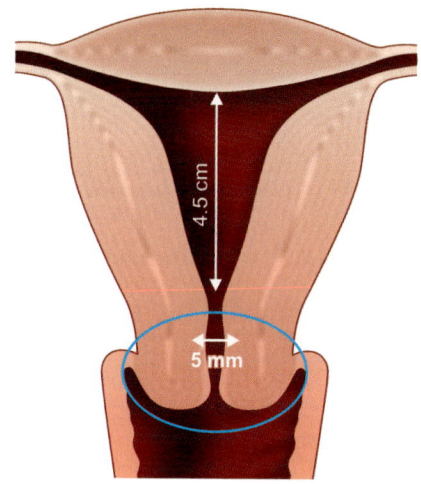

Fig. 3.3: Dimensions of uterus

Any hysteroscopes or resectoscopes with outer sheath diameter up to 5 mm are called miniaturized instruments. They are less invasive, less painful and without the need of cervical dilatation (Flowchart 3.2).

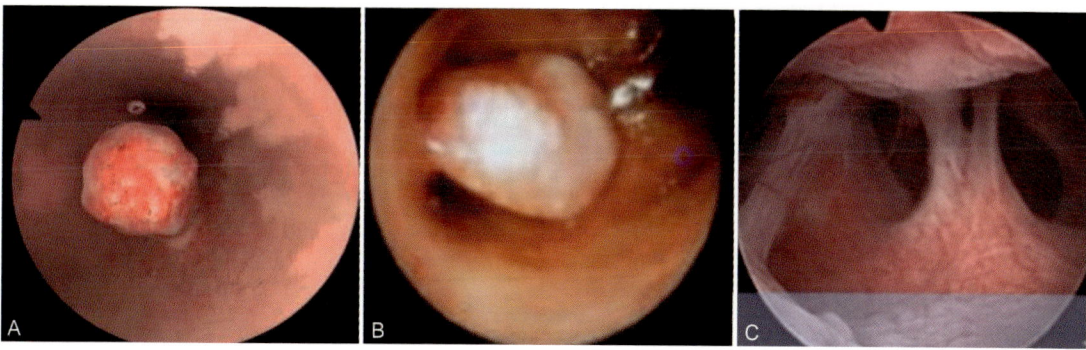

Fig. 3.2A to C: (A) Polyp; (B) Submucous myoma G0,1; (C) Intrauterine adhesions

Flowchart 3.2: Miniaturized instruments

Miniaturized intruments options*
Diagnostic
EndoSee™ office hysteroscope
Diagnostic and operative
• Bettocchi integrated office hysteroscope (BIOH)
• CAMPO trophyscope
• Bettocchi 5 mm hysteroscope
Office endometrial ablators
• Minitouch endometrial ablator
• Minerva endometrial ablation system
• Lina librata
• Mara water vapor ablation treatment
Office resectoscopes
Gubbini mini resectoscope
Hysteroscopic morcellators
• Truclear
• MyoSure

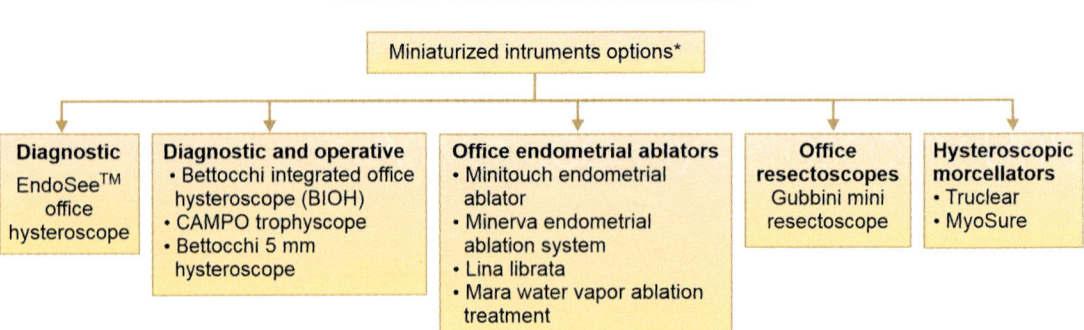

**Described in detail in chapter "innovations in hysteroscopy"*

4. Vaginoscopy

In 1997, Steffano Bettocchi introduced the **No touch entry technique** called "Vaginoscopy" (Flowchart 3.3). It is atraumatic insertion of hysteroscope into os, as **no** speculum or tenaculum is used.

To reduce the possible trauma during this phase, keep the scope located in the middle of the canal, avoiding stimulation of the muscle fibers (Fig. 3.4)

Flowchart 3.3: Vaginoscopy technique

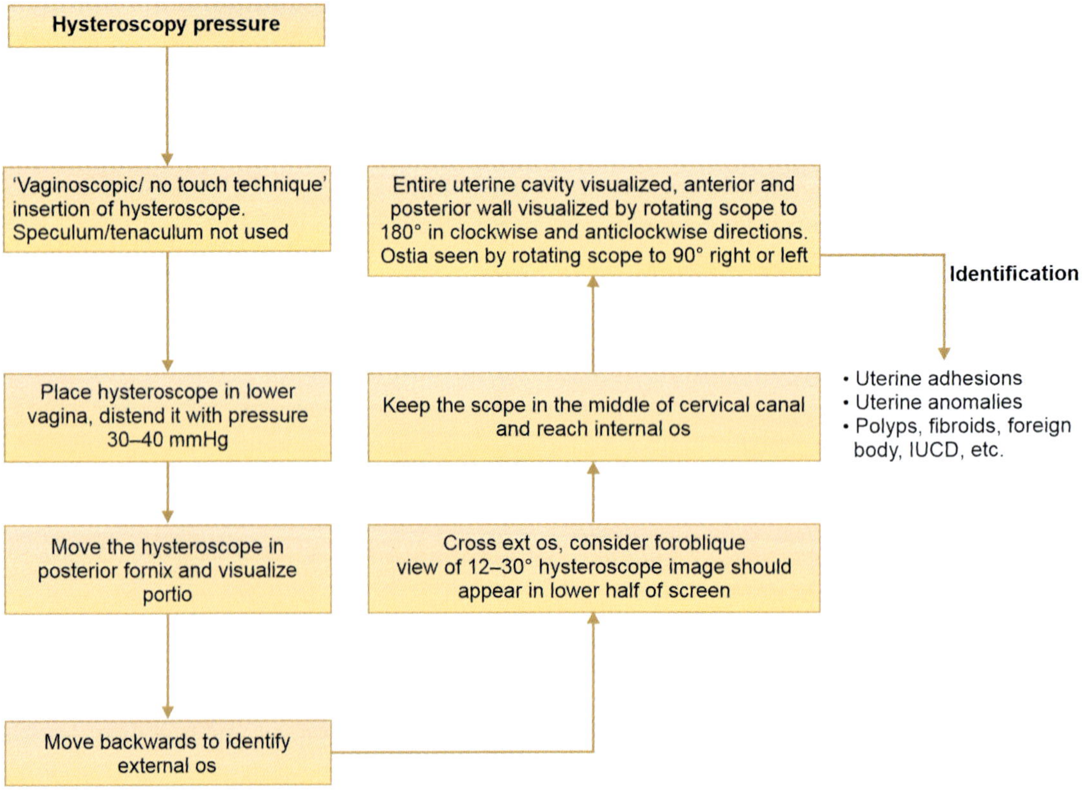

Hysteroscopy pressure
'Vaginoscopic/ no touch technique' insertion of hysteroscope. Speculum/tenaculum not used
Place hysteroscope in lower vagina, distend it with pressure 30–40 mmHg
Move the hysteroscope in posterior fornix and visualize portio
Move backwards to identify external os
Cross ext os, consider foroblique view of 12–30° hysteroscope image should appear in lower half of screen
Keep the scope in the middle of cervical canal and reach internal os
Entire uterine cavity visualized, anterior and posterior wall visualized by rotating scope to 180° in clockwise and anticlockwise directions. Ostia seen by rotating scope to 90° right or left
Identification
• Uterine adhesions
• Uterine anomalies
• Polyps, fibroids, foreign body, IUCD, etc.

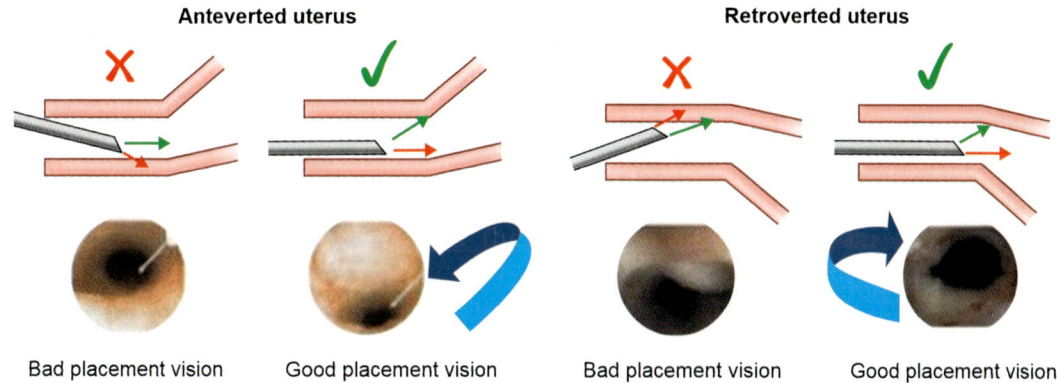

Anteverted uterus   **Retroverted uterus**

Bad placement vision   Good placement vision   Bad placement vision   Good placement vision

Fig. 3.4: Correct entry technique

Advantages of vaginoscopy

- Vaginoscopic approach consumes equal time as conventional approach
- Detailed evaluation of the vaginal walls, fornices, and ectocervix is obtained.
- Reduces patient discomfort, to a large extent
- Allows the examination, even in virgin patients, severe vaginal atrophy or stenosis.

5. Distension with Normal Saline is Preferred in Office Hysteroscopy

- Well tolerated and more comfortable for the patient
- Vaginoscopic approach is much easier with water distension medium
- Cost-effective
- Provide a superior and clearer hysteroscopic view in case of intrauterine bleeding.

Complications

- Pain (Table. 3.1)
- Bleeding
- Uterine trauma—laceration or perforation
- Failed hysteroscopy—cervical stenosis

Pain Sensation

Sensitive innervations of the uterus are present at myometrium, serosal surface and only basal thirds of endometrium (Fig. 3.5)

- *Upper vagina, cervix, and lower segment:* Parasympathetic fibers S2 to S4, forming Frankenhauser or uterovaginal plexus, that enters the uterus following the cardinal ligaments.
- *Body and fundus:* Sympathetic fibers— T10 to L2 via inferior hypogastric plexus, enters through utero-sacral ligaments and infundibulopelvic ligament, forming ovarian plexuses.

Table 3.1: Reasons for pain and measures to overcome	
Reasons for pain	**How to overcome?**
Speculum or tenaculum usage	No touch technique
Cervical dilation	Miniaturization of equipment
Passage of the hysteroscope through the cervical canal	Correct entry technique
Distension of the uterus with fluid	**Analgesia may be needed**
Operative procedures that damage the lower thirds of endometrial walls, e.g. endometrial biopsy, polypectomy or myomectomy, ablation or tubal sterilization	

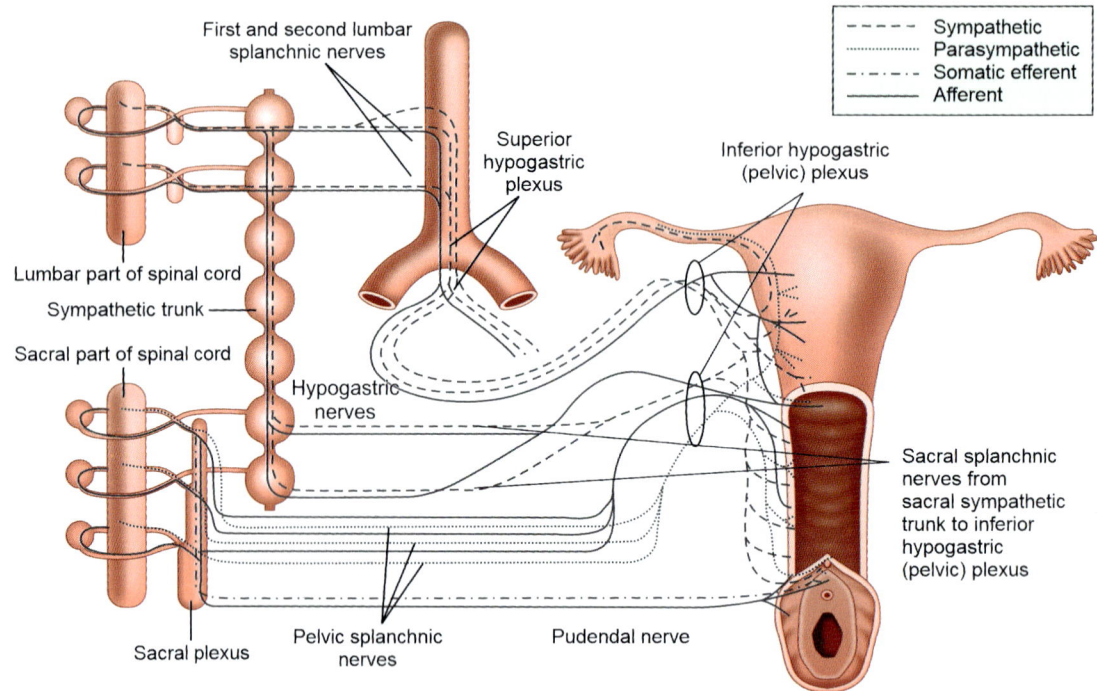

Fig. 3.5: Pain innervations of the uterus

- *Myometrium and basal third of endometrium:* Innervated by endomyometrial plexus.

Most literature suggests that office hysteroscopy in experienced hands is a well-tolerated technique and requires the use of analgesics only in selected patients.

Adequate patient selection—fundamental step to achieve a successful OH.

Factors Associated with Increased Pain

- Nulliparity
- Postmenopausal
- History of dysmenorrhea or chronic pelvic pain
- Anxiety
- Procedure > 15 mins *(30% more risk of pain when procedures exceed 3 minutes)*
- Endometrial polypectomy of polyps (>2.2cm) and duration of the procedure (more than 15 min) are the limiting factors.
- High distension pressure—optimal filling pressure for adequate visualization without causing excessive pain at 40–50 mmHg.

There are consistent good-quality evidence of a clinically meaningful difference in safety or effectiveness between different types of pain relief compared with each other or with placebo or no treatment in women undergoing outpatient hysteroscopy

Recommendations for Analgesics— Diagnostic Office Hysteroscopy

RCOG 2011: Tablet ibuprofen 400 mg or paracetamol 1 gram or any analgesic at least 1 hour before the procedure.

ACOG 2018

- Tablet misoprostol (off label) 200–400 micrograms oral or intravaginal, the night before surgery
- Preoperative NSAIDS
- Anti-anxiety medications.

Recommendations for Analgesics— Operative Office Hysteroscopy

- Para-cervical injections of local anesthetic significantly reduced pain in women undergoing outpatient hysteroscopy. Maximum dose of lidocaine is 4.5 mg/kg. 200 mg of lidocaine (20 ml of 1% lidocaine) is injected at cervicovaginal junction- 2.4.6.8.10 o'clock positions at 1.5–2 mm depth (Fig. 3.6)

- Combined cervical block protocols for the resection of polyps and myomas. Randomized trial found a statistically significant difference in pain score between a group receiving **paracervical and intracervical** block than the group receiving only intracervical block *(1.3 vs. 2.1, respectively)*
- Conscious sedation (0.25 mg IV fentanyl + 0.5 mg atropine + 2 mg midazolam)

Does not cause significant differences in terms of intraoperative or postoperative pain or the woman's satisfaction. Close monitoring is needed, as it can depress the CNS and has the potential to impair respiration, circulation or both. Thus it is not recommended.

Uterine Trauma

Lacerations to the cervix or uterine perforation Incidence: 0.002–1.7%

This complication has been drastically reduced due to the use of small-diameter endoscopes (outer sheath diameter under 5.5 mm) and vaginoscopy (entry under direct vision)

Factors associated

- Blind dilatation—cervical stenosis
- Tortuous cervical canal (e.g. fibroids)
- Deviated uterine cavity (e.g. acute flexion, pelvic adhesions, fibroids).

Overpassing Cervical Stenosis

Cervical stenosis is defined as cervical scarring of a variable degree, and comprising both subjective impression of narrowing and the completely obliterated external or internal os (Fig. 3.7).

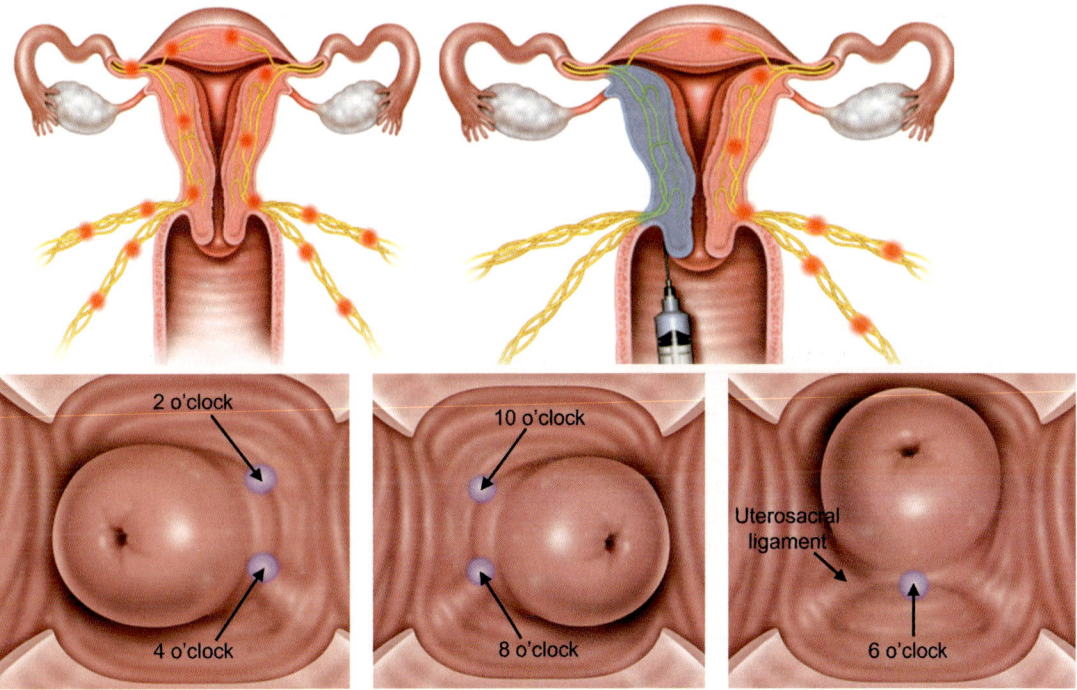

Fig. 3.6: Paracervical block technique

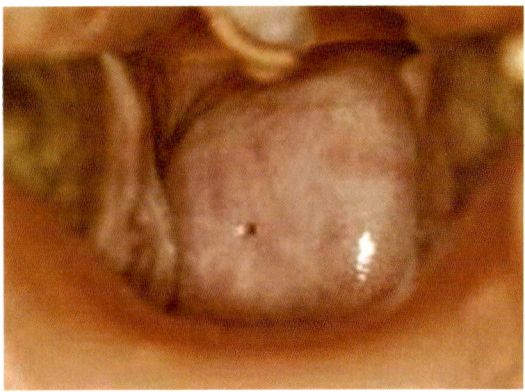

Fig. 3.7: Cervical stenosis

Etiologies: Postmenopausal atrophy, cervical surgery, previous caesarean section, nulliparity.

Medical methods

- Misoprostol 400 mg either orally or vaginally 6–8 h prior to surgery or 400 mg sublingually 2–4 h prior to surgery.
- Hygroscopic dilators—Lamineria tents or Dilapan S (3 × 55 mm or 4 × 55 mm) 12 hr before procedure
- Intracervical injection of vasopressin solution (4 IU in 100 cc sodium chloride) injected at the 4 and 8 o'clock positions.

Surgical methods

No sensitive nerve terminals or blood vessels have been demonstrated in the fibrous tissues, so it can be cut or recommended analgesics may be given.

5F (Karl Storz, Tuttlingen, Germany) mechanical instruments, e.g. forceps or scissors, may be used to overcome stenosis of the cervical channel in the office-based setting—*without causing any pain or bleeding.*

Moderate Stenosis

Fibrous ring may be cut at 2–3 points using sharp scissors or stretched by grasping forceps inserted within it with the jaws closed and then gently opened (Fig. 3.8A and B).

Severe Stenosis

Allows only the possibility to insert a needle-like bipolar electrode in order to cut the fibrotic ring of the EUO by creating 3–4 radial incisions, at 3 o'clock, 6 o'clock, 9 o'clock, and 12 o'clock positions (Fig. 3.8C).

Why Consider Office Hysteroscopy?

Gynecologist's Point of View

- Significantly better in diagnosing endometrial abnormalities compared to transvaginal ultrasound (TVUS) and saline infusion sonohysterography (SIS).
- Gold standard in assessing AUB in postmenopausal women.
- Dramatically reduces false-negatives associated with blind biopsies

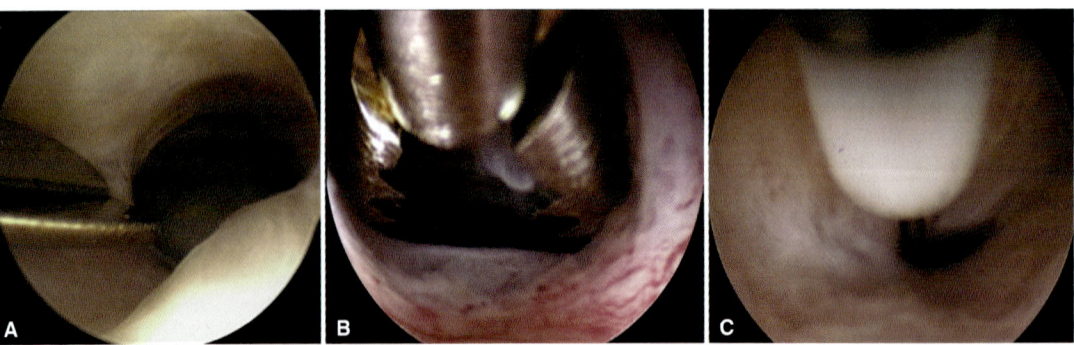

Fig. 3.8A to C: Overpassing cervical stenosis

Patient's point of view

- Cost effective
- Significant economic savings to patients in comparison to hospital (facility) procedures.
- Patients may not be subjected to potential dangers of general anesthesia.
- Number of office visits required to diagnose and treat intrauterine pathology and days off from work is reduced
- Patient has the option of watching their procedure in real-time which may increase a feeling of comfort.

✍ Key Points

1. OH is a commonly performed investigation; it is safe and of short duration.

2. Most women are able to have the procedure in an outpatient setting, with or without local anaesthesia, and find it convenient and acceptable.

3. Women must be offered, the choice of having the procedure performed as a day care procedure under general or regional anesthesia.

4. It is important that the procedure to be stopped, if a woman finds the outpatient experience too painful for it to be continued. Which may be at the request of the patient or nursing staff in attendance, or at the discretion of the clinician performing the investigation.

5. Successful OH is when, a women recommends it to *others-too*.

BIBLIOGRAPHY

1. American College of Obstetricians and Gynecologists. ACOG technology assessment in obstetrics and gynecology no. 13: hysteroscopy. Obstet Gynecol. 2018; 131: e151–e156.
2. Cooper NA, Khan KS, Clark TJ. Local anaesthesia for pain control during outpatient hysteroscopy: systematic review and meta-analysis.BMJ. 2010;340:c1130.1.
3. doi:10.1016/j.fertnstert.2010.03.047. 3. Soguktas S, Cogendez E, Kayatas SE, Asoglu MR, Selcuk S, Ertekin A. Comparison of saline infusion sonohysterography and hysteroscopy in diagnosis of premenopausal women with abnormal uterine bleeding. European Journal of Obstetrics and Gynecology and Reproductive Biology. 2012;161(1):66–70.
4. Grimbizis GF, Tsolakidis D, Mikos T, et al. A prospective comparison of transvaginal ultrasound, saline infusion sonohysterography, and diagnostic hysteroscopy in the evaluation of endometrial pathology. Fertility and Sterility. 2010;94(7):2720–2725.
5. Lau WC, Tam WH, Lo WK, Yuen PM. A randomised double-blind placebo-controlled trial of transcervical intrauterine local anaesthesia in out patient hysteroscopy.BJOG. 2000;107: 610e613.32. Kabli.
6. Lukes AS, Roy KH, Presthus JB, Diamond MP, Berman JM, Konsker KA. Randomized comparative trial of cervical block protocols for pain management during hysteroscopic removal of polyps and myomas.Int J Womens Health. 2015;7:833e839.
7. Munro MG, Brooks PG. Use of local anesthesia for office diagnostic and operative hysteroscopy. J Minim Invasive Gynecol. 2010;17:709e718.
8. RCOG/BSGE Joint Guideline, Green-top Guideline No. 59 March 2011 Best Practice in Outpatient Hysteroscopy.

Distension Media Problems: Fluid Overload and its Management

Rahul Manchanda, Aayushi Rathore

Hysteroscope was first introduced by Bozzini in 1807. Initially, contact hysteroscopy was performed to visualize the uterine cavity but it stimulated intrauterine bleeding which led to obscuration of view. This instigated the use of distension medium for adequate visualization of the cavity. Heinberg (1914) commenced the use of irrigation system during hysteroscopy. Attempts were made using gase (CO_2) as well as fluid distension media. In due time, the complications associated with their use were identified, one of which was fluid overload.

TYPES OF FLUID DISTENSION MEDIA

The characteristic features of an ideal distension media are that it should be isotonic, nontoxic, hypoallergenic and non-hemolytic. It should provide clear visualization of the uterine cavity and at the same time should be rapidly cleared from the body (Fig. 4.1 and Table 4.1).

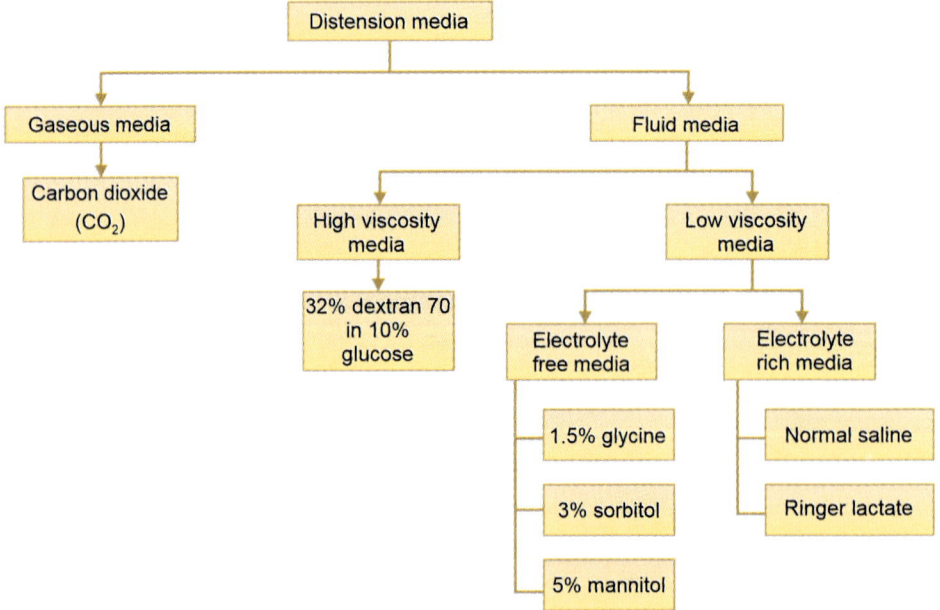

Fig. 4.1: Types of distension media

Table 4.1: Advantages and disadvantages of fluid distension media		
Type of fluid	**Advantages**	**Disadvantages**
Electrolyte free fluid		
• Glycine 1.5% • Sorbitol 3% • Mannitol 5%	• Can be used with monopolar energy devices	• Excessive absorption causes hyponatremia, hyperammonemia, and decreased serum osmolality with the potential to cause seizures, cerebral edema and death
Electrolyte rich fluid		
• Normal saline (NS)	• Easily availability • Hypoallergenic • Nontoxic • Inexpensive • Isotonic • Can be used in diagnostic and operative hysteroscopy • Can be used in cases with, mechanical laser, or bipolar energy sources	• Although the risk of hyponatremia and decreased serum osmolality can be reduced by using these media, pulmonary edema and congestive heart failure can still occur. • Careful input and output fluid monitoring is required

Incidence of Fluid Overload

The actual incidence of fluid overload varies according to the type of fluid being used in the surgery as well as the type of procedure being performed. It has been reported to be 0.1–0.2% in most of the studies.

AAGL 2013, BSGE 2016, ACOG 2018 defines fluid overload at following threshold deficit (Table 4.2).

Table 4.2: Threshold levels for various types of fluid distension media in hysteroscopy		
Distension media	**Healthy individuals**	**Elderly and compromised individuals**
High viscosity	500 mL	300 ml
Low viscosity hypotonic media	1000 mL	750 ml
Low viscosity isotonic media	2500 mL	1500 ml

Pathophysiology and Systemic Effects of Fluid Overload

Hemodynamic effects

Excessive fluid intravasation during hysteroscopy gives rise to hypervolemia which can manifest with symptoms ranging from mild dyspnoea and uneasiness to features of frank pulmonary edema. Pulmonary edema usually occurs when the serum sodium concentration falls below 100 mmol/L along with hypo-osmolality. This is often followed by a hypokinetic phase which presents with symptoms of low cardiac output such as hypotension. This occurs subsequent to natriuresis, osmotic diuresis and intracellular shift of water.

Cardiovascular

Heart failure and cardiovascular collapse can precipitate either due to hyperdynamic circulation because of fluid overload or due to depressed conductivity in the heart and bradycardia which can sometimes occur secondary to fluid overload. ECG changes in this scenario include depression of ST segment and T wave, prolongation of PQ interval and a wide QRS complex.

Vascular effects

The most common feature of fluid overload includes dilutional hyponatremia which occurs due to reduction of serum osmolality.

15–25% patients, develop excess fluid intravasation that is associated with a transient hyperkalemia of due to intracellular entry of irrigation fluid solutes. Dilutional hypoproteinemia can occur by 40–50% in severe cases. Additionally, metabolic acidosis develops with serum pH that ranges between 7.10 and 7.25.

Cerebral effects

Excessive fluid intravasation produces intracellular shift of water along the concentration gradient in the brain cells and subsequently development of cerebral edema, cerebral herniation and death. It occurs more frequently in premenopausal females due to inhibition of Na^+/K^+ ATPase pump by estrogen, which is responsible for maintaining the fluid balance inside the brain. Also, estrogenic inhibition of this pump in the myometrium increases the risk of absorption of fluid causing fluid overload. The peculiar feature of glycine overload is hyperammonemia and its associated encephalopathy in which case, the patient develops depressed consciousness, confusion and coma. Other features of glycine overload includes visual disturbances at concentration of 5–8 mmol/L, nausea, vomiting and abdominal pain at 10 mmol/L and heart failure, pulmonary edema and death between 21 and 80 mmol/L.

Complications of Fluid Overload
Electrolyte free media

1. **Asymptomatic hyponatremia:** Dilutional hyponatremia is initially asymptomatic when sodium concentration is >125 mOsm/L.
2. **Symptomatic hyponatremia:** Symptoms of hyponatremia begin when sodium levels fall below 125 mOsm/L which includes headache, nausea, vomiting and generalized weakness. As the levels fall below 120 mOsm/L there is confusion, lethargy, seizures, coma, arrhythmias, bradycardia and respiratory arrest.

3. **Cerebral symptoms:** As the fluid intravasation increases, it causes further decline in plasma osmolality and consequently an increase in the intracranial pressure and cerebral edema as described above. The symptoms include agitation, confusion, weakness, visual disturbance, blindness and headache which can eventually progress to cause brainstem herniation and even death.
4. **Excess sorbitol** intravasation causes hyperglycemia and hypocalcemia and the patient can present with myoclonus within an hour of the procedure. RBS monitoring should be done in such cases and if found to be increased, sliding scale insulin can be started. Calcium correction is done by infusion of 3 gm calcium gluconate over 10 min after taking advice from interventionist.

Electrolyte rich media

The incidence of hyponatremia is minimal while using normal saline, however, hypervolemia can manifest as pulmonary edema and heart failure. Hence, input–output monitoring of fluid coming out of hysteroscope is still necessary while using electrolyte rich media like normal saline for irrigation.

Impact of Anesthesia on Fluid Overload and Electrolyte Balance

It has been affirmed that fluid absorption is more under general anesthesia in comparison to paracervical block with 1% lignocaine and sedation (480 ml vs 253 ml). Additionally, there is a fall of sodium by more than 10 mOsm/L in case of use of general anesthesia. But these findings cannot be generalized due to short duration of procedures done under local anesthesia.

Prevention

Prevention is the best strategy to prevent complications related to fluid overload during hysteroscopy. The various strategies that can be employed are as follows:

1. Protocol should be made to respond to fluid overload
2. Thresholds should be predetermined considering the type of distension media used and the procedure being performed.
3. Strict input output monitoring should be done by a dedicated person in the operating room.
4. Use of automated delivery systems wherever feasible.
5. Error due to overfill of ~150 ml while using 3 L fluid bags should be considered
6. All three output sources should be included in calculation of fluid deficit (return from hysteroscope, spill from vagina and loss on the floor).

Treatment

Multidisciplinary approach is required for management of fluid overload which includes anesthetist, physician and interventionist with availability of HDU/ICU. Visual disturbances and hypertension are transient symptoms and they improve spontaneously in majority of the cases with supportive measures. Mild symptoms like nausea and vomiting requires treatment with antiemetics. Strict input–output monitoring should be done and fluid balance should be maintained. Earlier fluid restriction was advocated but there are several studies which show that plasma volume expansion should be done as stopping the irrigation can lead to development of sudden hypotension.

Electrolytes (Na^+, K^+ and Ca^{++}) and SpO_2 monitoring should be done and correction instituted accordingly. Specific management of hyponatremia and correction with 3% hypertonic saline at the rate of 1–2 mmol/L/hr is recommended till the level of 130 mmol/L is achieved. Rapid correction of hyponatremia is avoided as it can lead to central pontine myelinosis.

Management of Fluid Overload
(Table 4.3 and Flowchart 4.1)

If signs and symptoms are suggestive of heart failure and pulmonary edema, 2D echo and CXR are done and treatment with diuretics (IV 40 mg furosemide) should be initiated promptly. It should be avoided in cases where the patient is hemodynamically unstable to prevent development of hypotension and aggravation of hyponatremia. Diuretics should not be routinely used in all cases of fluid overload.

Cardiovascular collapse can be reversed if immediate intervention is done. Treatment of bradycardia and hypotension with atropine, adrenergic drugs and intravenous calcium is started to prevent mortality and morbidity.

Additionally, surgical management by retroperitoneal drainage of excess fluid has been reported by studies and can be undertaken only in case of massive absorption of fluid to reduce the mortality and morbidity.

Table 4.3: Management of hyponatremia	
Hypovolemic hyponatremia	**Management**
Asymptomatic hyponatremia and [Na^+] ≥120 mmol/L	• Fluid restriction (e.g. <1 L/day) • Loop diuretics, e.g. 40 mg furosemide (in case of suspected pulmonary edema)
Symptomatic hyponatraemia and [Na^+] <120 mmol/L	• Hypertonic (3%) saline (1 L=513 mmol/L NaCl compared with normal saline where 1 L=154 mmol/L) • Supplemental oxygen • Indwelling urinary catheter • HDU/ICU care • Multidisciplinary team involvement

Flowchart 4.1: Management of fluid overload

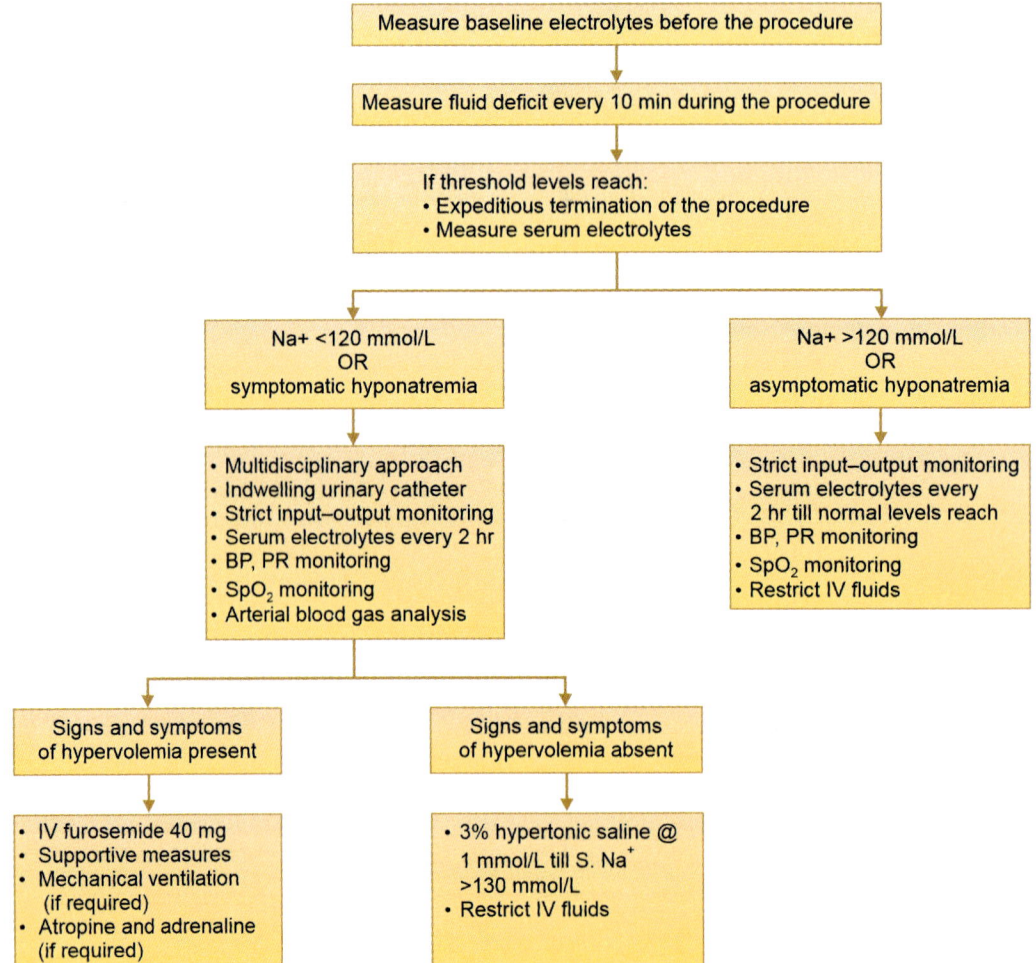

✍ **Key points**

1. Incidence of fluid overload is 0.1–0.2%

2. Distension of uterine cavity during hysteroscopy can be done by using either high viscosity media or low viscosity media.

3. Low viscosity media are further categorized as electrolyte rich media (normal saline) and electrolyte free media (3% sorbitol, 1.5% glycine and 5% mannitol)

4. Electrolyte free media are commonly associated with dilutional hyponatremia and features of hypervolemia including cerebral edema, heart failure and pulmonary edema.

5. Electrolyte rich media are less frequently associated with dyselectrolytemia, but cardiac failure and pulmonary edema can occur due to hypervolemia.

6. Integrity of myometrial vessels, intrauterine pressure, duration of surgery, size of the uterus and physical characterstics of the fluid media used determines the risk of fluid overload .

7. Intrauterine pressure should always be kept below the MAP to prevent excessive fluid intravasation

8. Use of automated fluid delivery system is recommended

9. Strict input–output fluid monitoring should be done in all cases of hysteroscopy

10. Surgeon should be able to recognize the signs and symptoms of fluid overload in its initial stages, as prompt intervention can reduce the morbidity and mortality

11. Multidisciplinary approach is required for management of fluid overload

12. Symptomatic hyponatremia should be corrected slowly using hypertonic saline (3%)

13. Diuretics should be reserved for cases with heart failure and pulmonary edema as it can precipitate hypotension and could further decrease sodium concentration by causing natriuresis

BIBLIOGRAPHY

1. AAGL Practice Report: Practice Guidelines for the Management of Hysteroscopic Distending Media: (Replaces Hysteroscopic Fluid Monitoring Guidelines. J Am Assoc Gynecol Laparosc. 2000;7:167–168.). J Minim Invasive Gynecol. 2013 Mar-Apr;20(2):137–48.

2. ACOG Technology Assessment No. 13: Hysteroscopy. Obstet Gynecol. 2018 May;131(5):e151–e156.

3. BSGE/ESGE guideline on management of fluid distension media in operative hysteroscopy. Gynecol Surg. 2016; 13(4): 289–303.

4. Hahn RG. Fluid absorption in endoscopic surgery. Br J Anaesth. 2006 Jan;96(1): p8–20.

5. Taskin O, Buhur A, Birincioglu M, et al. Endometrial Na1, K1-ATPase pump function and vasopressin levels during hysteroscopic surgery in patients pretreated with GnRH agonist. J Am Assoc Gynecol Laparosc. 1998;5: 119–124 (Evidence I).

6. Valle RF. Development of hysteroscopy: from a dream to a reality, and its linkage to the present and future.J Minim Invasive Gynecol. 2007 Jul-Aug;14(4):407–18.

Modalities to Reduce Volume of Systemic Fluid Absorption (Preoperative and Intraoperative)

Richa Sharma, Rahul Manchanda

At the time of hysteroscopy, the fluid which is used to irrigate the cavity can get absorbed into the systemic circulation and excess of this intravasation can cause symptoms of fluid overload and other associated complications.

The various mechanisms which have been postulated for fluid absorption are as follows:

1. **Integrity of venous sinuses:** Uterine myometrium is enriched with venous sinuses, the integrity of which will prevent systemic absorption of fluid, especially during diagnostic hysteroscopy. However when there is resection of this myometrium in operative hysteroscopy procedures like myomectomy, metroplasty and endometrial resection, these vascular sinuses are damaged and the distension fluid gains access to systemic circulation in increasing quantity which can give rise to fluid overload. This mechanism is particularly important in procedures requiring extensive resection of the endometrium and myometrium.

2. **Intrauterine pressure (IUP):** For systemic absorption of intracavitatory fluid, the pressure inside the uterine cavity needs to rise above the mean arterial pressure (MAP) for the fluid to enter these vessels. The risk of fluid overload is directly proportional to the intrauterine pressure

during the hysteroscopy procedure. When the MAP is low, lower intrauterine pressures can also exaggerate the risk of fluid overload. Moreover, extra caution needs to be exercised in elderly patients and those with cardiovascular or renal co-morbidities.

3. **Duration of surgery**: With an increase in the duration of surgery, the risk of fluid absorption increases and hence the duration of surgery during hysteroscopy should be kept to a minimum to prevent complications.

4. **Size of the uterine cavity:** Large surface area of uterus can increase risk of fluid absorption. Moreover, the duration of surgery also increases with the size of the cavity increases due to more surface area. However, on the other hand, larger intra-uterine pressure is required to exceed the threshold for fluid overload.

Absorption of the irrigation fluid used during hysteroscopy can be reduced by the following preoperative and intraoperative interventions:

Preoperative Measures
1. Choice of distension media

The type of distension media used should be such that, least amount of complications occur in case of its excess absorption. The type of procedure to be performed, instruments (monopolar/bipolar/mechanical) used during surgery and the physical characteristics of fluid should be considered while choosing the type of distension media.

2. GnRH analogue

Use of GnRH analogue preoperatively decreases the fluid deficit (more in pre-menopausal females) by its action on Na^+/K^+ ATPase pump and consequently dec-reases the morbidity and mortality associated with fluid overload.

Intraoperative Measures

   i. **Intracervical vasopressin:** Injection of intracervical vasopressin immediately before dilatation causes vasoconstriction of the myometrial vessels and sub-sequently cause less systemic fluid absorption during surgery. However, it can also induce cardiovascular collapse, myocardial infraction and death. So, anesthetist should always be made aware while its instillation and maxi-mum concentration of <0.4U/Ml should be used to prevent these complications.

  ii. **Intrauterine pressure:** Intrauterine pressure should always be maintained below the mean arterial pressure during hysteroscopy preferably between 70 and 100 mmHg (depending on the size of the uterus, muscle thickness and tone). For short procedures, 40 mmHg intrauterine pressure is recommended. It is pos-tulated that the control of intrauterine pressure leads to decreased absorption of fluid by 85%.

 iii. **Delivery system:** Use of automated fluid delivery system during hysteroscopy is presently advocated which monitors the fluid deficit and intrauterine pressure in real time and alerts the surgeon about risk of excess fluid intravasation.

  iv. **Technique of resection:** It also influences the risk of fluid overload as the risk is less when vaporizing electrodes are used in comparison to cutting loops.

   v. **Duration of surgery:** The duration of hysteroscopy should be kept minimum.

✍ Key Points

1. Integrity of myometrial vessels, intrauterine pressure, duration of surgery, size of the uterus and physical characterstics of the fluid media used determines the risk of fluid overload
2. Threshold of fluid deficit differs in healthy individuals in comparison to elderly and patients with renal or cardiovascular com-promise
3. Threshold of fluid deficit also varies according to the type of media used.
4. Choosing appropriate distension media is crucial in prevention of fluid overload.
5. Preoperative use of GnRh analogue also helps in decreasing the fluid deficit along with its role in reduction of intraoperative blood loss.
6. Intracervical injection of vasopressin just prior to cervical dilatation causes vasoconstriction of myometrial vessels and decreases fluid deficit
7. Intrauterine pressure should always be kept below the MAP to prevent excessive fluid intravasation.

BIBLIOGRAPHY

1. Chudnoff S, Glazer S, Levie M.Review of vasopressin use in gynecologic surgery. J Minim Invasive Gynecol. 2012 Jul-Aug;19(4):422–33.
2. Corson SL, Brooks PG, Serden SP, et al. Effects of vasopressin administration during hystero-scopic surgery. J Reprod Med. 1994;39:419–423.
3. Parazzini F, Vercellini P, De Giorgi O, Pesole A,Ricci E, Crosignani PG. Efficacy of pre-operative medical treatment in facilitating hysteroscopic endometrial resection, myo-mectomy and metroplasty: literature review. Hum Reprod 1998;13:2592–7.
4. Phillips DR, Nathanson HG, Milim SJ, et al. The effect of dilute vasopressin solution on blood loss during operative hysteroscopy: a rando-mized controlled trial. Obstet Gynecol. 1996; 88:761–766.

Monitoring Fluid Deficit

Richa Sharma, Rahul Manchanda

A variety of fluid media delivery systems have been developed over time which began with the use of simple gravity systems that delivers the fluid by hydrostatic pressure. The height of the fluid column affects the intrauterine pressure in gravity fed systems. At the height of 1–1.5 m, the intrauterine pressure achieved is ~ 70–100 mmHg. Later, delivery systems evolved and fluid was infused using pressure cuffs around the delivery bag to maintain a constant flow in the uterus and to limit obscuration of view by the blood, mucus and debris. However, this endangered the risk of excessive fluid intravasation as the intrauterine pressure was often more in this case.

This prompted the idea of development of automated delivery system which provides better control over input–output monitoring and which displays the intrauterine pressure and fluid deficit in real time. These systems are equipped with alarm systems which alerts the operating surgeon about the increased risk of fluid overload when necessary. Some of these automated pumps also titrate the intrauterine pressure and keeps it in the appropriate range. Nonetheless, these pumps are costly and are especially useful when used in long and complex procedures (Fig. 6.1).

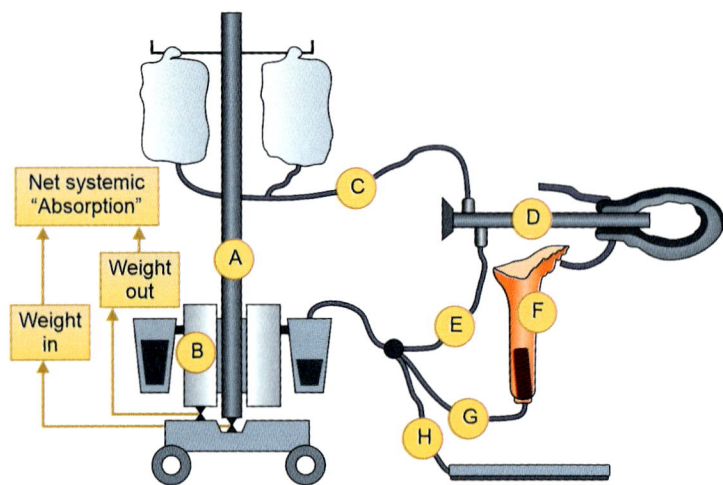

Fig. 6.1: Mechanism of action of automated fluid management systems (A to H see text)

Mechanism of action of automated fluid management systems: The infusion media is placed on the pole (A). The outflow canisters are attached to a separate collection platform (B). The fluid is infused through tubing (C) into the resectoscope (D). Outflow fluid is evacuated via tubing (E) into the collecting canisters. Fluid that leaks around the resectoscope is collected by a specially designed pouch (F) or, if it falls on the floor, by a door mat, each of which are connected to the collecting canister with tubing (G and H). The microprocessor subtracts the collected fluid (weight out) from the infused fluid (weight in) to calculate the fluid balance and the net systemic absorption.

Types of Fluid Deficit Monitoring

There are two kinds of hysteroscopy systems: open system and closed system. For calculation of fluid deficit, the amount of fluid entering the hysteroscopy system and the amount of fluid leaving, it should be calculated precisely and accurately.

- **Open system:** Fluid escapes out through the cervix onto the drapes and the floor making accurate monitoring difficult and brings about errors in calculation of fluid deficit.
- **Closed system:** The fluid returns via suction tubing into the outflow canister and thus accurate measurement of outflow fluid is feasible. Also specially designed drapes, floor mats and collection bags are commercially available to remove errors in the calculation of outflow. Fluid escaping from the usual surgical drapes is likely to be missed from measurement and this accounts for overestimation of fluid deficit. Error also occurs in calculation of fluid deficit because of ~3–6% overfill of inflow bag which should be taken into consideration while calculation. Moreover, if there is significant bleeding during the procedure, it can add up to the outflow volume and generates false low

deficit value. Automated closed hysteromats, e.g. Storz and Olympus are most ideal (Fig. 6.2A and B).

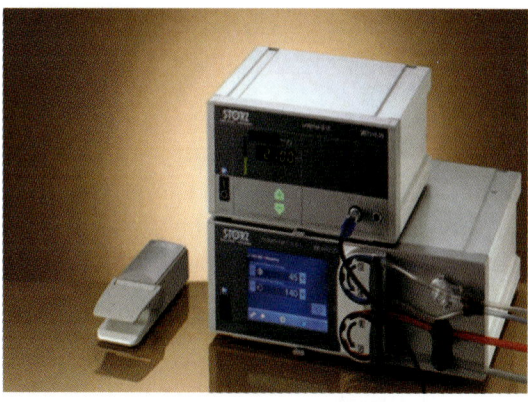

Fig. 6.2A: Karl Storz EASI hysteromat

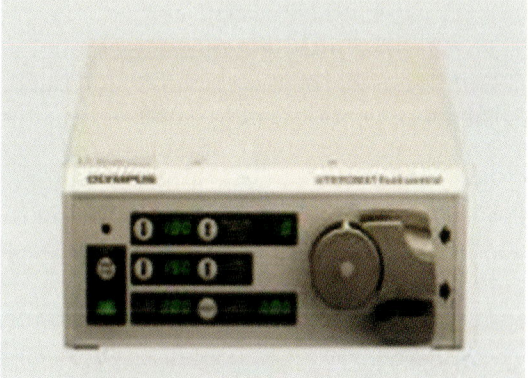

Fig. 6.2B: Olympus automated hysteromat

Methods to Measure Fluid Balance

1. *Volumetric fluid balance calculation:* In this technique, the difference between inflow and outflow fluid volumes is calculated by either manual methods or by automated pumps. However, errors can occur and hence it is unreliable.

2. *Gravimetry method:* The patient is operated on a bed scale and the body weight is measured. The difference in the body weight of the patients gives an estimation of the amount of fluid absorbed during the procedure. However, the amount of blood loss and the volume of intravenous fluid

given to the patient should also be taken into consideration while using this method to avoid errors.

3. *Central venous pressure monitoring:* Central venous pressure rises by 2 mmHg for every 500 ml intravasation of fluid in the circulation. As the gravimetry method, this method is also influenced by the amount of blood loss and intravenous fluid received and hence is not reliable.

4. *Isotope measurement:* It is considered the most accurate and sensitive method to detect even low grade fluid absorption. These tracers are added to the irrigating fluid and their plasma concentrations determine the amount of fluid intravasation. However, due to the concerns regarding their safety of use, these are not routinely used clinically.

5. *Ethanol:* The principle of using ethanol is the same as that of tracer isotopes. Although, its concentration can be analysed using breath-analysers during surgery which makes it easier to use. In this technique, 1% ethanol is used and concentration of more than 75 ml per 10 min of surgery indicates fluid overload.

6. *Electrolyte measurement:* Hypervolemia leads to dilutional hyponatremia and decreased sodium concentration measured intraoperatively indicates excess fluid intravasation .

A running measurement of fluid deficit should be made every 10 min during the procedure and when each bag finishes. A dedicated OT room personnel should be assigned the role of monitoring the inflow–outflow from the hysteroscopy systems, calculation of fluid deficit and its communication to the operating surgeon.

According to ACOG 2018 technology assessment guidelines on hysteroscopy, intravenous fluid monitoring has been given key importance. It states that intravenous fluids should also be monitored and taken into account to prevent fluid overload in patients, in addition to intrauterine fluid monitoring. It further reinforces that the threshold of fluid deficit should be less in elderly patients and those with cardiovascular or renal co-morbidities and caution should be exercised in such cases.

BSGE 2016 guidelines recommend to use a especially designed proforma during operative hysteroscopy for documentation and monitoring of fluid deficit (Fig. 6.3).

✍ Key Points

1. Automated fluid measurement systems provides constant surveillance on fluid deficit and pressure.
2. Fluid deficit balance must be recorded every 10 min and at the end of each fluid bag used.
3. BSGE 2016 guidelines recommend use of proforma during operative hysteroscopy for documentation and monitoring of fluid deficit
4. Two kinds of hysteromet systems: Open system and closed system.

BIBLIOGRAPHY

1. AAGL Elevating Gynecologic Surgery. AAGL Practice Report: Practice Guidelines on Intrauterine Adhesions Developed in Collaboration With the European Society of Gynaecological Endoscopy (ESGE). J Minim Invasive Gynecol. 2017;24 (5):695–705.
2. AAGL Practice Report: Practice guidelines for the management of hysteroscopic distending media. JMIG 2013;20:137–148.
3. ACOG Technology Assessment No. 13: Hysteroscopy. Obstet Gynecol. 2018 May; 131(5):e151–e156.
4. BSGE/ESGE guideline on management of fluid distension media in operative hysteroscopy. First published: 21 June 2018.https://doi.org/10.1111/tog.12503.
5. BSGE/ESGE guideline on management of fluid distension media in operative hysteroscopy. Gynecol Surg DOI 10.1007/s10397–016–0983–z. Published online 6th Oct 2016.
6. Hahn RG. Fluid absorption in endoscopic surgery. Br J Anaesth. 2006 Jan;96(1):8–20.
7. Polyzos MP, Mauri D, Tsioras S. Intraperitoneal dissemination of endoemtrial cancer cells after

Date _____

Operation _____

Surgeon _____

Anaesthetist _____

Energy of resectosocpe _____

Fluid medium used _____

Method of limiting intrauterine pressure:

Gravity	height above patient _____ meters
Pressure bag	maximum pressure used _____ mmHg
Automated system	brand _____

Method of monitoring distension fluid in theatre

Sole person identified to monitor fluid deticit, measuerd every 10 min	yes ☐	no ☐
Drape used with fluid reservoir	yes ☐	no ☐
Closed system, i.e. fluid collection with suction	yes ☐	no ☐

Operation start fine	Fluid inpout	Fluid output	Fluid balance
+10 min			
+20 min			
+30 min			
Review: If not likely to complete procedure in under 60 min consider stopping			
+40 min			
+50 min			
Review: Consider stopping procedure at 60 min			
Length of procedure	Final	Final	Final
Min			
STOP procedure if fluid deficit reaches 1000 ml Hypotonic solution (750 ml if elderly or with co-morbidities) or 2500 ml isotonic solution (1500 ml if elderly or with co-morbidities)			

Fig. 6.3: BSGE/ESGE recommended inflow and outflow chart

hysteroscopy. A systematic review and meta-analysis. Int J Gynecol Cancer 2010;20:231-267.

8. Taskin O, Buhur A, Birincioglu M, et al. Endometrial Na1, K1-ATPase pump function and vasopressin levels during hysteroscopic surgery in patients pretreated with GnRH agonist. J Am Assoc Gynecol Laparosc. 1998; 5:119–124 (Evidence I).

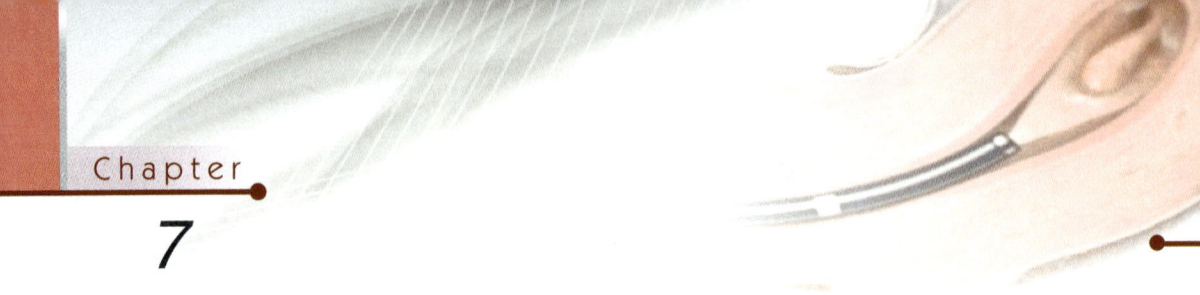

Advanced Hysteroscopy Unit

Sushma Deshmukh

Hysteroscopy has pioneered the process of endoscopic viewing of uterine cavity with less invasive form of treatment. Step by step the operative hysteroscopic procedures have revolutionized the therapeutic aspect of gynecological surgeries. Advanced hysteroscopy unit has become a vitally important unit in the armamentarium for the management of many day-to-day clinical problems as well as in difficult situations giving rewarding results. Actually modern hysteroscopy represents a technological triumph achieved by many known and unknown scientists who spent sleepless nights and put lifetime efforts. Nowadays, hysteroscopic surgery is pivotal in the management of many gynecological pathologies.

Most of the diagnostic hysteroscopy procedures are performed in the office or clinic, whereas operative hysteroscopy is usu-ally performed in an OR (operative room) or hospital surgicenter. Detailed history, physical examinations and routine investigations are must to minimize complications. The success of hysteroscopy depends on the choice of anesthesia, choice of distension media, the instrumentation, and the experience of the surgeon. As hysteroscopy has increasingly become the method of choice for treatment of intrauterine pathology, there is need to update hysteroscopy unit with safety measures.

ADVANCED HYSTEROSCOPY UNIT

Whenever we think about advanced hystero-scopy unit, the upgradation should be from the place (OR), instruments–equipments, ancillary systems, surgeon, surgeries and techniques. Advanced hysteroscopy Unit (AHU) often necessitates teamwork that involves medical-nursing expertise working within the sphere of gynecologic endoscopy in an institution and technical support. It also involves the patient and her feedback. This should be updated continuously with learning lessons from other institutions. It is also necessary to involve different specialities of endoscopic surgery with interchanging national and international experience.

ADVANCED HYSTEROSCOPY UNIT COMPONENTS (AHU)

1. Efficient team (Flowchart 7.1)
2. Well furnished operation room
   - Prefabricated modular OT/integrated operation room
   - Hydraulic table with comfortable stirrups.
   - Mobile cart containing monitor, camera unit with recording system, light source with fiberoptic cable, pressure pump and electrosurgical unit.

Flowchart 7.1: Efficient team

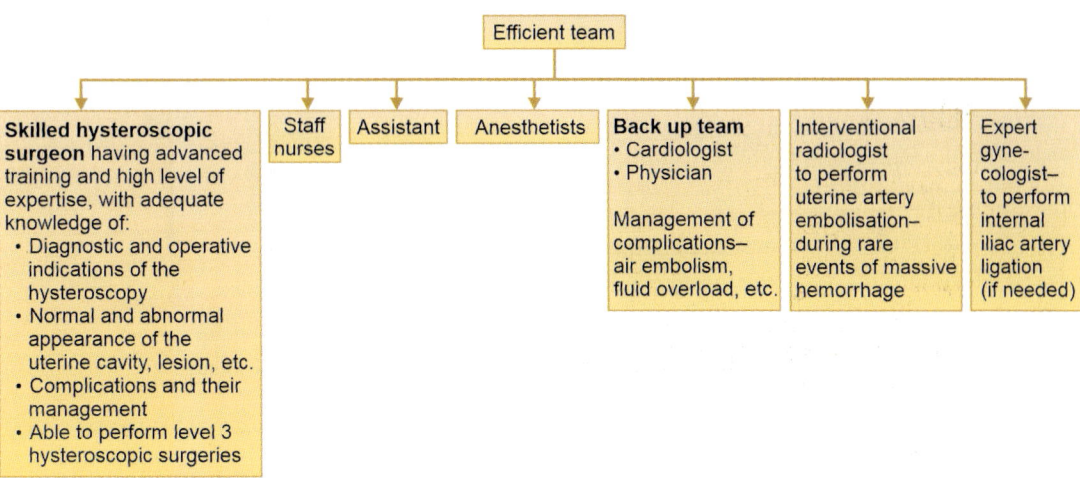

3. Basic and advanced instruments (Telescopes and sheaths with operative instruments):
   • Office instrument set
   • Operative instrument set
   • Resectoscope with all electrodes
   • Newer advanced instruments
4. Mandatory use of BSGE/ESGE 2016 safety checklist proforma for monitoring fluid management during operative hysteroscopy.

Operating Room

An organized and well-equipped operating room (OR) is essential for successful hysteroscopy procedures which includes prefabricated modular operation theatres instead of older OR suites for endoscopy. As these AHU modules are made of steel coatings, they provide antibacterial, antifungal and antialgal features for long and safe run. All the walls in the OR should have smooth surfaces (no visible joint) and absence of sharp edges which prevent any chance of accumulation of stagnant air or builds up of contamination. Most of the hysteroscopic units are combined with laparoscopic units giving comprehensive care. OR with laminar air flow, ceiling mounted pendants, theater control panel, seamless flooring, hermetically scaling sliding doors, X-ray viewing screen, scrub station, pressure stabilizers, electronic touch panel, etc. are the features of modern laparoscopic OR suite. Leading endoscopic equipment and instrument have developed integrated OR system which gives the surgeon, ability to control the equipment virtually, by "touch" technology or radio remote control over the entire OR. These systems make up for the total remodelling of existing OR. All pieces of equipment and lighting are ergonomically mounted from ceiling booms and equipment settings can be precustomized to be readied for different surgeons and procedures as required.

In OR (Fig. 7.1), the mobile cart, OT table, trolley anesthesia machine, should be arranged in proper order (Fig. 7.2).

Hydraulic Table with Comfortable Stirrups

Nowadays we get very nice automated OT tables which are made friendly for anesthetists as well as doctors. The surgeon should know and confirm all the facilities of it. The table should be easily operable and have the capabilities for Trendelenburg and

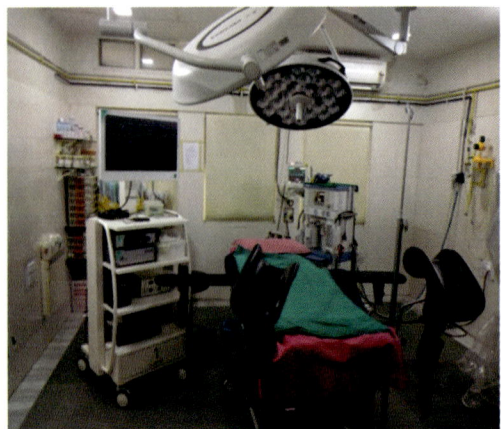

Fig. 7.1: Operation room

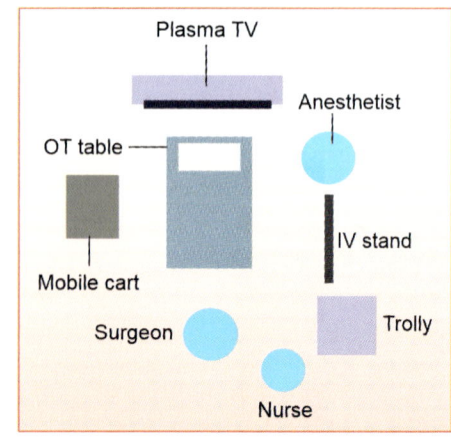

Fig. 7.2: Proper OT arrangement in hysteroscopy

reverse Trendelenburg in automated fashion for associated laparoscopy. Modern stirrups are optimally padded and have gel inserts that hold and support the knees, calves, and ankles permit prolonged procedures and minimize pressure and nerve injuries. Additionally stirrups should have the capability for altering the position of lower extremities during the procedure by compressing the lever at the bottom of stirrup handle (Fig. 7.3).

Position of the Patient

Hysteroscopy is performed in a modified dorsal lithotomy position; the patient is supine, and the legs are held in stirrups. A correct lithotomy position is necessary, i.e. with legs apart supported in leg rests with the buttocks at the edge of the table or few centimetres extending beyond the table. Back should be flat to avoid postoperative back strain. Avoid extreme flexion, abduction and lateral rotation of the hip.

Position of the Surgeon

The surgeon sits between the patient's legs. The eye level of the patient and surgeon should match. But in acutely anteverted uterus, the surgeon's chair should be at lower level and in acutely retroverted at a higher level. Some surgeons will prefer standing

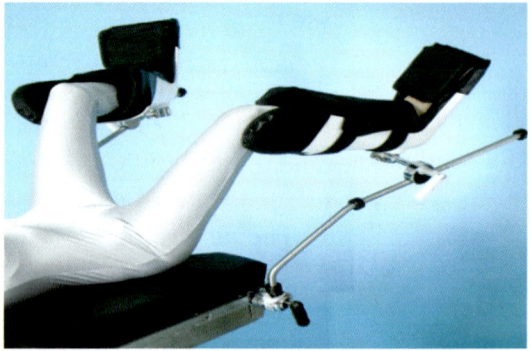

Fig. 7.3: Lithotomy bars with stirrups

position. In that case the camera and the telescope should be at or just below the lower border of umbilicus. In a sitting position the whole system should be at few inches above the level of umbilicus.

Choice of Anesthesia

- **Verbal method:** In this method, the main aspect is counselling of patient. It can be done by doctor or staff nurse. Thorough explanation of the procedure is given to the patient. During procedure patient is to be engaged in talking or patient can listen the music by head phones. In modern units of hysteroscopy most of the procedures are with very small diameter instrument and without any local or general anesthesia.

- **Local anesthesia:** The administration of local anesthesia in hysteroscopy can be topical, intrauterine, intracervical, and paracervical. Safe use of anesthetic drugs requires a complete understanding of the potency, avoiding toxicity, and early recognition of potential complications.

- **Systemic medications:** Nonsteroidal anti-inflammatory drugs (NSAIDs), opioids, Benzodiazepines, misoprostol being used by many doctors. Misoprostol has been studied and being used for cervical ripening prior to hysteroscopy, specially in nulligravida and operative hysteroscopy like resection.

- **General or regional anesthesia:** In operative hysteroscopy like resection of submucous myoma, isthmocele we prefer general anesthesia.

Mobile cart containing monitor, camera unit with recording system, light source with fiberoptic cable, pressure pump and electrosurgical unit (Fig. 7.4)

With all the various options available, it becomes confusing for a novice about what to buy. For example, the camera system will not be solely dedicated for hysteroscopy use but also will be used for laparoscopy also.

Hence a system which will be useful for both should be bought.

Gadgets of Hysteroscopy

Distension Media

To view the uterine cavity we need distension medium. There are various types of media (gas as well as liquid) like CO_2 gas, high viscosity 32% dextran 70 and low viscosity fluids, including glycine, sorbitol, saline. A pressure of 45 mmHg or higher is generally required for adequate distension of the uterine cavity. Generally pressure should not exceed the mean arterial pressure (70–100 mm) to minimize extravasation.

Nowadays normal saline is used as distension media when bipolar current is used which has given opportunity to use it in more advanced and complex procedures. Some surgeons prefer to use monopolar current. For standard operative hysteroscopy with monopolar resectoscopes, low viscosity, non-conductive fluids such as 1.5% glycine, is used most often because there are no electrolytes to disperse the current and impede the electrosurgical effect. Hysteropump, i.e. endomat (Fig. 7.5) which allows monitoring of irrigation and suction pressure and controls flow rate. Normally, the settings

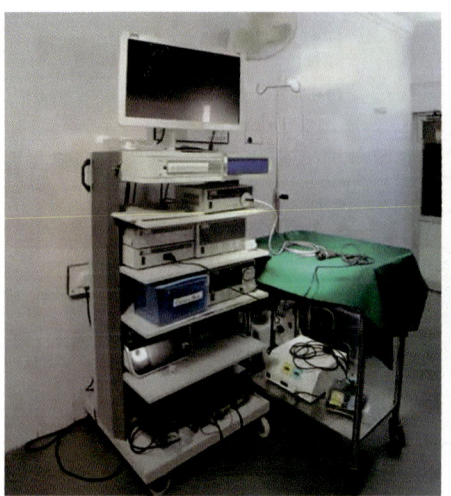

Fig. 7.4: Mobile cart containing

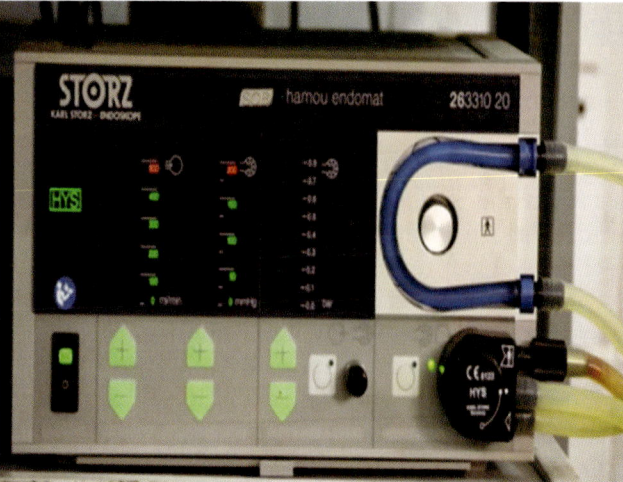

Fig. 7.5: Endomat pressure pump

are kept at 75 mmHg inflow and 0.25 bar suction and a flow rate of 200 mL/mt.

Normal saline is a useful and safe medium for diagnostic and operative procedures utilizing laser, mechanical instruments or bipolar electrosurgical devices. Even if there is absorption of a substantial volume of solution, saline does not cause electrolyte imbalance. Therefore, saline is a good fluid for minor as well as major procedures performed in the office.

Newer hysteromat from Storz Hysteromat endoscopic automatic system irrigation (EASI) is touch screen operated and has various modes such as automatic, manual, high pressure mode, coagulation, blood mucous mode. Also can be used for laparoscopy (Fig. 7.6).

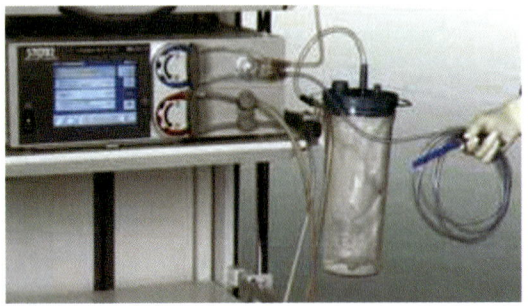

Fig. 7.6: EASI

Light Source and Light Cable (Fig. 7.7)

Light delivery inside the uterus is an important feature for proper image generation. The intensity of the light should be bright enough to illuminate the entire uterine cavity at the same time there should be no undue glare and heat production. The technical specifications of cold light source have a major impact on the image quality. A good quality light source with a xenon lamp will give good illumination. Light is transmitted though fiberoptic or fluid light cables with a diameter of 3.5–5 mm and a length of 180–350 cm for standard hysteroscopy procedure. The xenon generator provides

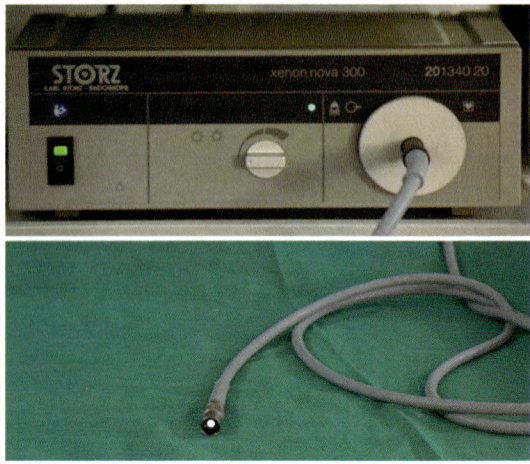

Fig. 7.7: Light source and light cables

white light, which gives a superior color and intensity. Because it runs from a standard 110 volt or 220 volt wall outlet, the light source requires no special electrical connections.

Recording System and Camera (Fig. 7.8)

It is very important to record each procedure. No system is complete without digital imaging and data capture. It will allow image or video captured during operation to be assessed, edited, printed and saved on disk for documentation. It is also important for

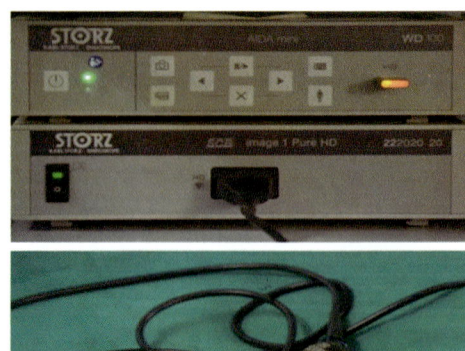

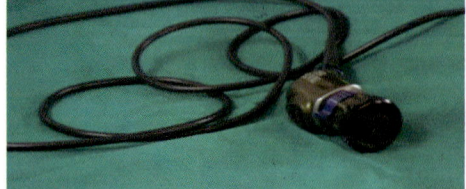

Fig. 7.8: Camera and recording system

distant learning and interactions. Different types of video cameras are available. The image quality depends on resolution and sensitivity.

Modern HD (high definition) camera offers very high resolution and almost natural color inside the uterine cavity. HD camera has proved to be really superior to the earlier innovations in the camera systems and has improved the vision greatly. Complete systems with video recorders are available.

The newer top line camera systems come with *"dialog light control"* (communication between the light source and the camera), the camera and light source are interconnected through a separate cable and the camera controls the light volume automatically in the "dialog" mode. This gives the optimum image quality with maximum protection for patients and equipment.

Optical Systems

There are two main optical systems, i.e. (1) direct and (2) contact.

The direct optical hysteroscope provides the surgeon with a global view of the uterine cavity. A distending medium is used and the image is well illuminated and has excellent contrast and resolution. Conversely, contact hysteroscopes work without a distending medium and provide only a focal view of the endometrial cavity. Thus, unless the uterine cavity is explored in a slow, systematic fashion, significant pathology can be missed. This approach is rarely used.

Electrosurgical Unit and Electrodes

Modern high frequency (HF) electrosurgical units can be operated both in monopolar and bipolar mode. Electrosurgical instruments use household current that is transformed into radiofrequency current. Monopolar instruments use current that flows from an active electrode, through tissue, having a cutting or coagulating effect. Current travels through the patient, exiting by way of a return electrode plate (usually placed on the patient's thigh) to the electrosurgical unit. In the bipolar system, the electrical arc is formed around the loop itself and is passed through the tissues only between the two ends of the loop.

For bipolar cautery, normal saline is used as a distension medium. For monopolar current glycine, sorbital used as distension medium. Current recommendation is to use the electrolytic fluids in diagnostic cases which can be easily converted in operative procedure in the same sitting using mechanical, laser or bipolar energy. Or in planned operative cases we can directly use bipolar or laser energy. Since they conduct electricity, these fluids should not be used with monopolar electrosurgical devices.

Medical Display Monitor

Medical display monitors have unique requirements above conventional TV screens. Foremost amongst them is a higher resolution. These have stringent medical safety and quality criteria. The special features are: a secure and insulated electric circuit which is spill and splash proof. It also guards against electrical interference from the other electronic gadgets in the operation theater. It has ability to tile multiple monitors so that the same image is displayed on various monitors, image enhancement. It has antiglare and low reflection screens and support of multiple and simultaneous inputs with excellent grayscale performance. The monitor can be connected to recording and archiving devices.

Instruments (Telescopes, Sheaths and other Operative Instruments)

Instruments play key role in the hysteroscopic surgery. One has to be familiar with assembling the elements of the operative hystero-resectoscope with the power sources, uterine distending fluids. Also their possible complications and to be alert for any intraoperative or postoperative complications.

We can divide the instruments according the operative procedure. In current scenario there is no longer distinction between diagnostic and operative procedures but rather a single procedure in which the operative part is perfectly integrated with the diagnostic work up. So it can be either office hysteroscopy or operative hysteroscopy under anesthesia.

Office Hysteroscopy

To view the 'hystera' through hysteroscopy is like learning the philosophy of hystera, i.e. uterus. The hysteroscope is also designed in a delicate way to adjust the curves of uterus (Fig. 7.9) and occupy space in the uterus without disturbing its anatomy and physiology. That is why today most of the hysteroscopic procedures do not need anesthesia.

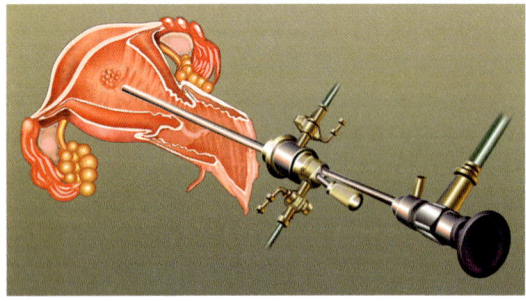

Fig. 7.9: Hysteroscope and uterine cavity

We can directly introduce the scope in the vagina without the speculum (i.e. vaginoscopy) and advance the scope further without any premedications or anesthesia to treat benign uterine pathologies (like endometrial polyp, septum, etc.)

'See and treat' is the password of office hysteroscopy.

There are many types of telescopes available.

- 2.9 mm Bettochi hysteroscope which is commonly used.
- 1.9 mm Bettochi hysteroscope
- 2 mm trophy scope

- Bettochi integrated office hysteroscope (BIOH)
- Versascope
- Endosee
- UBIPack GYN (SoproComeg, La Ciotat cedex, France)

2.9 mm Bettochi Hysteroscope

It can be used with a single flow operating sheath (4.3 mm) in combination with an outer sheath (5 mm) as a continuous flow operating system.

There are three main parts (Figs 7.10 and 7.11)

Bettocchi's forward: Oblique telescope 30°, diameter 2.9 mm, length 30 cm, Bettocchi's inner sheath, size 4.3 mm, with channel for semirigid 5 Fr operating instruments, Bettocchi's outer sheath 5 mm.

Office hysteroscopy introduces the concept of a single procedure in which, along with diagnostic work-up, the operative part is integrated according to need. Thus, along with the visualization of uterine cavity, one can take the biopsy or treat the benign intrauterine pathologies as a routine office procedure without anesthesia.

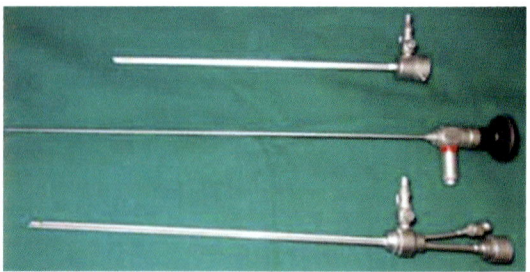

Fig. 7.10: Bettocchi's hysteroscope with three parts

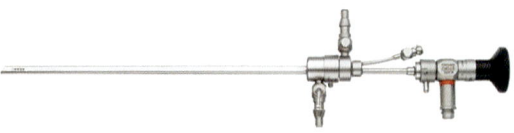

Fig. 7.11: Bettocchi's hysteroscope assembled with outer sheath of 5 mm

Bettocchi's 1.9 mm Hysteroscope

This newer version very much helpful for postmenopausal patients with cervical stenosis.

There are three main parts: Bettocchi's forward: Oblique telescope 30°, diameter 1.9 mm, length 30 cm, Bettocchi's inner sheath, size 3.6 mm, with channel for semirigid 5 Fr operating imnstruments, Bettocchi's outer sheath 4.2 mm

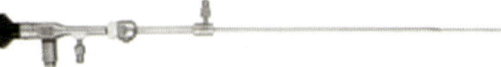
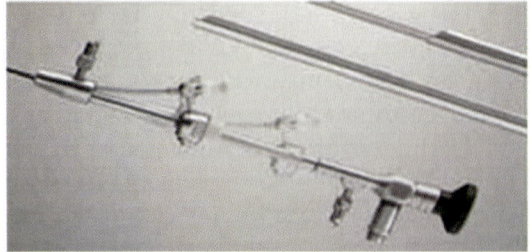

Fig. 7.12: Trophy scope

2 mm Trophy Scope

This is of new generation designed by Rudy Campo has an outer diameter of only 2.9 mm. with interesting characteristics: This hysteroscope (Fig. 7.12) has been named after the multicentre study TROPHY "Trial of outpatient hysteroscopy" for which it was designed. [TROPHY (trial of office hysteroscope) El-Toukhy T, Campo R, et al. Trial of Outpatient hysteroscopy [TROPHY] in IVF. Reprod Health 2009 Dec; 3 (6):20].

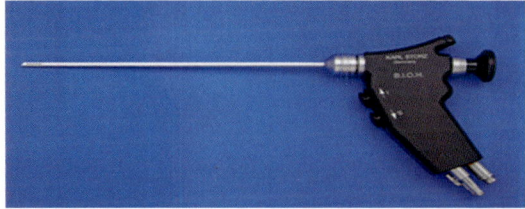

Fig. 7.13: Bettocchi Integrated office hysteroscope

Bettochi Integrated Office Hysteroscope (BIOH)

Bettocchi integrated office hysteroscope is a 2 mm 30° rod lens telescope ergonomically designed with continuous flow operative channel for 5 Fr instruments. Total diameter = 4 mm. Single handed operation and control of inflow and outflow (Fig. 7.13).

Flexible Versascope

Versapoint bipolar electrosurgical system has been developed as an alternative to the use of mechanical hysteroscopic instrument and the resectoscope. This is a telescope with external diameter of 1.8 mm, length 28 cm, providing 0° field of vision (Fig. 7.14A and B). It has outer disposable continuous flow diagnostic cum operative sheath of 3.5 mm with rotatable collar. The operating

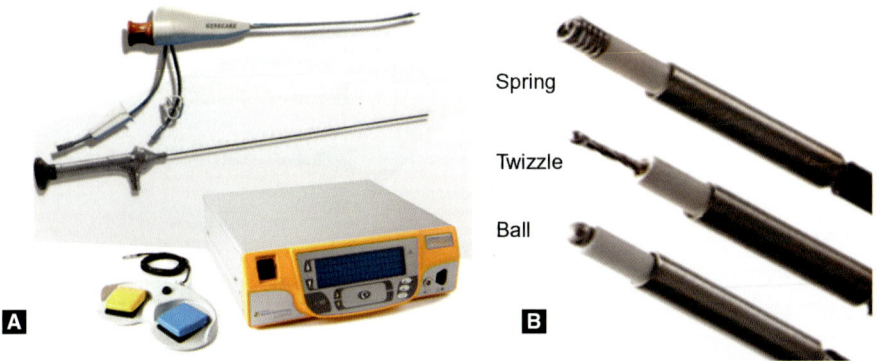

Spring

Twizzle

Ball

A　　**B**

Fig. 7.14A and B: Gynecare Versapoint™ bipolar electrosurgery system

channel has an expandable instrument channel which can easily accommodate instrument till 7 Fr diameter.

It consists of dedicated bipolar electro-surgical generator and two types of electrode: Twizzle, specifically for precise and con-trolled vapourization resembling cutting) and spring, indicated for diffuse tissue vaporisation. Each electrode consists of an active electrode located at the tip and a return electrode located on the shaft, separated by a ceramic insert.

UBIPack GYN **(SoproComeg, La Ciotat cedex, France)** is to provide a portable system for undertaking hysteroscopic procedures. Can be inserted into a USB port of a laptop or personal computer (Fig. 7.15). It is portable friendly unit.

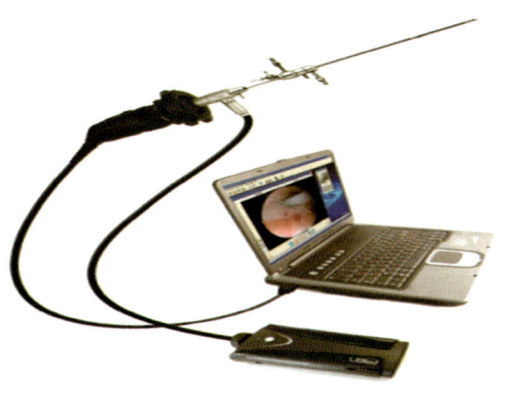

Fig. 7.15: UBIPack GYN

Mechanical Instruments

Most of the operative hysteroscopic instru-ments have a semirigid design and a dia-meter of 1.67 mm (5 French). There are many instruments used for office hysteroscopy but the main, which are required commonly are punch biopsy grasper, crocodile forceps and scissors (Figs 7.16 and 7.17)

1. Scissors

These scissors have one fixed and the other movable jaw- Semirigid, blunt, single action jaws, 5 Fr, length 34 cm. Another variety is pointed scissors.

2. Alligator Grasping Forceps

These forceps are helpful for remaining small polyps, foreign body, IUCD and endometrial biopsies. Semirigid, blunt, double action jaws, 5 Fr, length 34 cm.

3. Spoon Biopsy Forceps

Excellent for remaining small polyps and can be used for taking endometrial biopsy and can get a substantial tissue for biopsy.

4. Punch Biopsy Forceps

For resistant tissue biopsies such as from atrophic endometrium for myometrial biopsy.

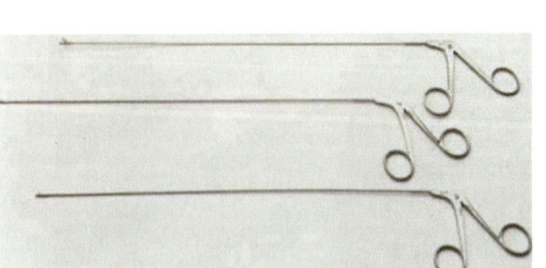

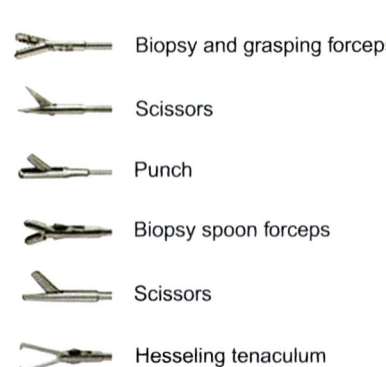

Biopsy and grasping forceps

Scissors

Punch

Biopsy spoon forceps

Scissors

Hesseling tenaculum grasping forceps

Figs 7.16 and 7.17: Mechanical instruments 5 Fr

5. Bipolar Dissection Electrode

Semirigid, 5 Fr, length 42 cm.

Operative Hysteroscopy

For operative hysteroscopy training sessions with experienced hysteroscopist are essential. Anesthetist will be needed for monitoring the patient and to keep patient comfortable. It is important to pay attention to proper assembly of equipment, distension fluids and its system, i.e. inflow and outflow, light source (xenon or LED) and connection to electrodiathermy unit, may it be monopolar or bipolar.

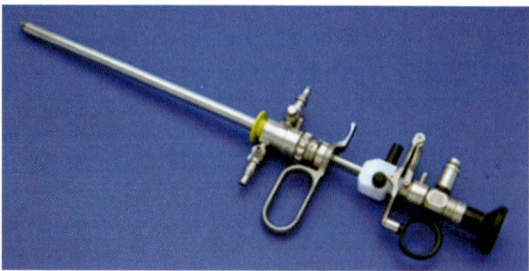

Fig. 7.18: Resectoscope—unipolar

Electrical Instruments

- Monopolar needle electrode
- Bipolar needle electrode
- Monopolar retracting loop for polypectomy
- Resectoscope

The resectoscope consists of a classic endoscope (Figs 7.18 and 7.20), with diameters ranging between 2.9 mm and 4 mm–preferably with a 12° or 30° viewing angle to keep the electrode within the field of view—combined with a cutting loop operated by a passive spring mechanism, and two sheaths for continuous irrigation and suction of the distension medium. Apart from the cutting loop (Fig. 7.19), other instruments such as Collin's knife and a variety of vaporizing or coagulating electrodes can be used with the working element of the resectoscope. There are various sets available. For 24 Fr inner and 26 Fr outer we use 4 mm telescope and for 19 Fr inner and 22 Fr outer we use 2.9 mm telescope.

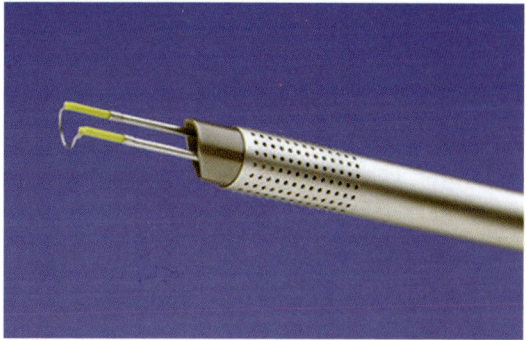

Fig. 7.19: Unipolar with cutting loop

Gubbini's Resectoscope

It is also very nice instrument that one should include in the list of resectoscopes. Many options are available for 2.9 mm telescope like 16 Fr inner/18 Fr outer (Gubbini midi), 14 Fr inner/16 Fr outer (Gubbini original), 14 Fr inner/16 Fr outer (Gubbini ellipse)

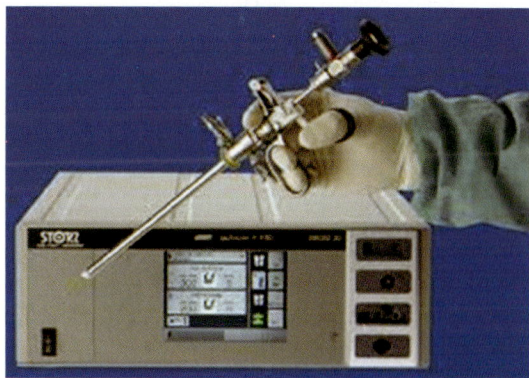

Fig. 7.20: Bipoar resectoscope

It is available in both unipolar and bipolar strength (Figs 7.21 and 7.22).

Laser

Nowadays, laser is used in hysteroscopy. (Fig. 7.23). Laser energy has the advantages in precision (Fig. 7.24) of tissue destruction that are not shared by the electrical energy. There are various types like diode, Nd:YAG laser. Light energy from lasers is transformed

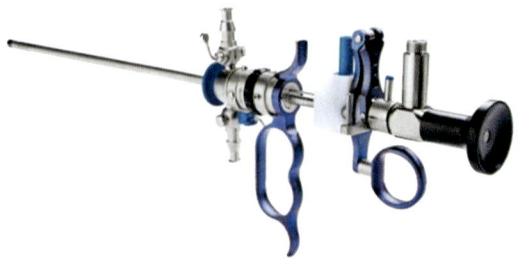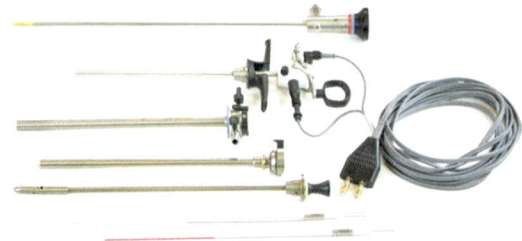

Figs 7.21 and 7.22: Gubbini's Resectoscope—assembled and disassembled

to thermal energy by electron flow. MyoFiber® and PolyFiber® are designed for tissue vaporization in polyps, septum, submucous myoma with the OPPIuM (office preparation of partially intramural myomas) successful technique (Fig. 7.24). The surgeon must be familiar with the physics governing the actions of lasers or electrosurgical tools and with the tissue actions exerted by these energized devices. Proper selection of patients depends on disease pathology and location. High power applied for a long period of time is risky, and will inevitably lead to unwanted tissue injury.

Hysteroscopic Morcellation

Invention of mechanical hysteroscopic morcellators has made a great improvement in management polyps and myomas. Hysteroscopic morcellator was developed to reduce problems of fluid overload, uterine perforation due to electric current, lack of visualization and need of removal of resected fragments resulting in a time-consuming procedure.

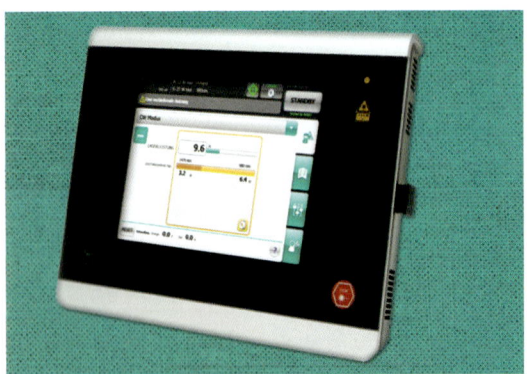

Fig. 7.23: Leonardo® dual 45 or 100 laser

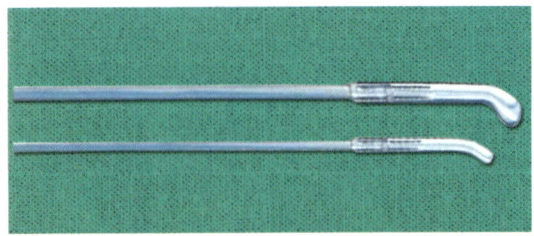

Fig. 7.24: MyoFiber® and PolyFiber®, designed for tissue (*Courtesy*: Dr Sergio Haimovich) vaporization in fibroids and polyps.

- Truclear™ 5.0 System (Smith and Nephew, London, UK) (Fig. 7.25) which was introduced in 2011 and for outpatient use, it has the distinct advantage of small size, with a 2.9 mm cutting blade and a 5.0 mm hysteroscope for office or ambulatory use with no or local anesthesia. Polyps, small myomas and retained products of pregnancy can be removed in that way.
- MyoSure® (Fig. 7.26) Tissue Removal System (Hologic, Marl-borough, USA) was introduced after the Truclear System. The MyoSure system is a fast, convenient way to remove intrauterine pathology, pairing direct hysteroscopic visualization with minimally invasive tissue resection.
- Intrauterine Bigatti Shaver introduced by Bigatti (Fig. 7.27)

Hysteroscopic morcellation devices introduced during the past decade may effectively treat intrauterine pathology, especially polyps and submucous fibroids. The

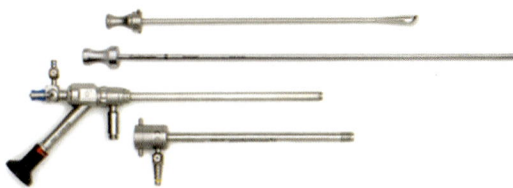

Fig. 7.25: Trueclear hysteroscope

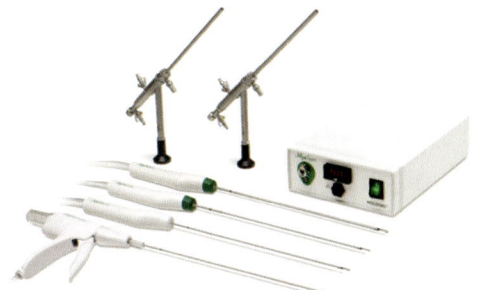

Fig. 7.26: MyoSure system

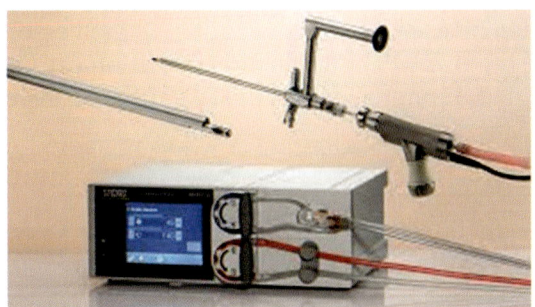

Fig. 7.27: Intrauterine Bigatti Shaver

smaller morcellators are suitable for use in an outpatient setting without need of anesthesia using normal saline as a distension media and with significantly faster time of procedure. However, hysteroscopic mechanical morcellators are not suitable for uterine leiomyomas type 1 and 2 because of their incapability to remove intramural component of tumor.

So the selection of surgery can be

- Mechanical by scissors, forceps
- Electrosurgical—monopolar resectoscope, bipolar standard electrode, bipolar versapoint Laser—ND: YAG.

Complications

In a tertiary centre we need to gear up to prevent and face all the complications. With proper OR set up, instrumentation, expert anesthesia back up, surgical skill and acumen we can prevent, minimize and tackle complications. The hysteroscopist should remember that in hysteroscopy, we are operating with a single hand with one instrument within one opening in a short time duration limit (Flowchart 7.2).

a. *Anesthesia Related:* Can be due to vasovegal or local anesthesia in office hysteroscopy due to general or regional anesthesia. To carry on high tech hysteroscopy surgeries we need proper anesthesia machines, OR set up and an expert anaesthetist.

b. *Position related:* To care about nerve injuries, avoid forced flexion and extreme external rotation. Proper lithotomy position should be given.

c. *Distension media:* Commonest complication occurs with distension media is fluid overload. It can occur with any liquid medium. With usage of non-ionic media (glycine-sorbitol) TCRE-like syndrome can occur. However, with saline also there can be fluid overload (hypervolemia). But office procedures with bipolar and saline as distension medium this complication is reduced. To prevent this, the input–output chart (fluid deficit chart) should be maintained. Nowadays, special lithotomy

Flowchart. 7.2: Complication of operative hysteroscopy

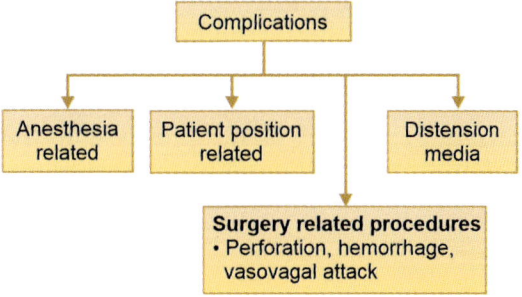

drapes with tubings at the lower end are there to calculate the fluid deficit.

d. *Surgery related procedures:* Perforation, hemorrhage, vasovagal attack, etc.

Uterine Perforation

Patients of severe cervical stenosis, nulligravida, postmenopausal patients are more prone for perforation. Immediate diagnosis is very important to avoid further complications like intestinal injury.

The surgeon should suspect perforation when there is inability to maintain proper uterine distension. Bleeding denotes that you are either in wrong plane or perforation. And one should stop the procedure. "Serosal Sign"—Imminent sign of uterine perforation, visualisation of abdominal contents, intestine, etc. are graver signs and should need immediate action.

Management

Uterine perforation with mechanical instruments like scissor or grasper or by hysteroscope along with sheath should be usually managed conservatively. But we need to admit the patient, fasting and monitoring of vital parameters for 24 hr. Sonography with complete blood count (CBC) to be done when needed. Watch for vomiting, abdominal distension and pain. It symptoms and signs worsen, then laparotomy is required.

Perforation with Electric Energy

Stop the flow and surgery and disconnect the electric cord of electrosurgical unit with hysteroscope. Simultaneous laparoscopy should be done. Place the hysteroscope near the area of perforation to inspect the bowel beyond uterus. Pelvis fills quickly with the distension media after perforation. Hysteroscope can even be placed through perforation

to yield an excellent view of the under surfaces of bowel immediately adjacent to injured area. If any doubt of visceral organ injury exploratory laparotomy should be performed.

Hemorrhage

This could be due to cervical tissue/vessel lacerations, deep myometrial vessel, myometrial blood vessel or intra-abdominal blood vessel injury.

Management

Stop the procedure and watch for the bleeding whether it is minimal or severe.

Find out the cause and assess it. If required put Foley catheter 25 cc balloon (4–24 hr), - Intrauterine pitressin soaked gauze or injection. If bleeding is due to vessel laceration in the myometrium then cautery can be used carefully to cauterize the vessel. Embolization/uterine artery ligation can be tried. Hysterectomy is the last option to save patient.

Gas Embolism

- Incidence 1:10,000–100,000.
- Types: Active and passive gas embolism.

It is a catastrophic event and if not diagnosed can lead to death of the patient complains of severe chest pain, dyspnea, oxygen saturation decreases.

Management

Stop the procedure on slight suspicion. Administer 100% oxygen. CPR/ionotropic drugs may be required. Anesthetist, OR staff including surgeon should work harmoniously.

So while dealing with the difficult cases as well as its complications, we really need advanced hysteroscopy unit. AHU is the need of today's modern technology.

✍ Key Points

1. Advanced hysteroscopic unit involves the upgradation should be from the place (OR), instruments–equipment, ancillary systems, surgeries and techniques.

2. Well furnished operating room with apt arrangements for hysteroscopy and proper instruments like monitor, camera unit with recording system, light source with fiberoptic cable, pressure pump and electrosurgical unit should be ready on the mobile cart.

3. The surgeon should have thorough knowledge of telescopes, various distension media, electrical surgical unit and electrodes. And he/she should be well versed with minor or major advanced techniques.

4. Current recommendations are for 'See and Treat' method of office hysteroscopy without anesthesia. We can treat many benign uterine pathologies like endometrial polyp, septum. One can manage 80% of the conditions with Bettocchi's 2.9 mm office hysteroscope. Various mechanical accessory instruments are there to carry out the procedures. Nowadays, we are having 1.9 mm Bettocchi's instrument.

5. **UBIPack GYN** is portable friendly unit for undertaking hysteroscopic procedures. It can be inserted into a USB port of a laptop or personal computer.

6. For conditions like fibroids, isthemocele we require resectoscope with electrical surgical unit and electrodes. There are various sets available. For 24 Fr inner and 26 Fr outer we use 4 mm telescope and for 19 Fr inner and 22 Fr outer we use 2.9 mm telescope.

7. Gubbini's resectoscope is also available. Many options are available for 2.9 mm telescope like 16 Fr inner/18 Fr outer (Gubbini midi),14 Fr inner/16 Fr outer (Gubbini original), 14 Fr inner/16 Fr outer (Gubbini Ellipse). It is available in both unipolar and bipolar strength.

8. Nowadays , laser is also used in hysteroscopy. Laser energy has the advantages in precision of tissue destruction that are not shared by the electrical energy.

9. Invention of mechanical hysteroscopic morcellators has made a great improvement in management polyps and myomas. Hysteroscopic morcellator was developed to reduce problems of fluid overload, uterine perforation due to electric current, lack of visualization and need of removal of resected fragments resulting in a time-consuming procedure. Truclear™, The MyoSure®, Bigatti Shaver.

10. In a tertiary centre we need to gear up to prevent and face all the complications. With proper OR set up, instrumentation, expert anesthesia back up, surgical skill and acumen we can prevent, minimize and tackle complications.

11. In dealing with the difficult cases as well as in complications we really need advanced hysteroscopy unit.

BIBLIOGRAPHY

1. Advanced Hysteroscopic Surgery Training-Mark M. Erian, MD, Glenda R. McLaren, MD, and Anna-Marie Erian, MD -JSLS. 2014 Oct–Dec; 18(4): e2014.00396.

2. Advanced Hysteroscopic Surgery: Quality Assurance in Teaching Hospitals-Mark M. S. Erian, DM (High Doctorate of Medicine), Glenda R. McLaren, MD, and Anna-Marie Erian, MD-JSLS. 2017 Apr-Jun; 21(2): e2016.00107.

3. Baggish MS.Contact Hysteroscopy:A new technique to explore the uterine cavity.Obstet Gynecol.1979;54:350.

4. Bettocchi S,Selvaggi L.A Vavinoscopic approach to reduce pain of office hysteroscopy.J Am Assoc Gynecol Laparosc 1997;4:255–8.

5. Bettochi S,Ceci O, Di Venere R, Pansini MV, Pellegrino A, Marello F, Nappi L Advanced operative office hysteroscopy without anesthesia: analysis of 501 cases treated with a 5Fr. Bipolar electrode. Hum Reprod.2002;17:2435–38.

6. Brill AI. Energy systems for operative hysteroscopy. Obstet Gynecol Clin North Am 2000; 27:317–32

7. Haimovich S, Mancebo G, Alameda FAgramunt S, Sole´-Sedeno JM, Hernández JL, Carreras R. Feasibility of a new two-step procedure for office hysteroscopic resection of submucous myomas: results of a pilot study. Eur J Obstet Gynecol Reprod Biol. 2013;168:191–4.

8. Hoekstra PT, Kahnoski R, McCamish MA, et al. Transurethral prostatic resection syndrome a new perspective: encephalopathy with associated hyperammonemia. J Urol 1983; 130:704–707.

9. Istre O. Fluid balance during hysteroscopic surgery. Curr Opin Obstet Gynecol 1997;9: 219–225.

10. Itzkowic DJ, Laverty CR. Office hysteroscopy and curettage.a safe diagnostic procedure. Aust N Z J Obstet Gynaecol 1990;30:150–153.

11. Manual of Operative Hysteroscopy. *AICOG* 2013;6–12.

12. Marana R, Marana E, Catalano GF. Current practical application of office endoscopy. Curr Opin.Obstet Gynecol 2001;13:383–7.

13. Phillips DR, Nathanson HG, Milim SJ, et al. The effect of dilute vasopressin solution on blood loss during operative hysteroscopy: a randomized controlled trial. Obstet Gynecol 1996; 88:761–766.

14. Pratice Committee of American. Society for Reproductive Medicine in Collaboration with Society of Reproductive Surgeons. Myomas and Reproductive Function. *Fertil Steril* Nov 2008; 9 (5 suppl); S125–30.

15. See and Treat hysteroscopy in daily practice-Attilio De Spiezo Sardo, Carmine Nappi pg. 11–23.

16. Thomas JA, Leyland N, Durand N, et al. The use of oral misoprostol as a cervical ripening agent in operative hysteroscopy: a double blind, placebo controlled trial. Am J Obstet Gynecol 2002;186:876–879.

17. Zupi E, Luciano AA, Valli E, et al. The use of topical anesthesia in diagnostic hysteroscopy and endometrial biopsy. Fertil Steril 1995; 63:414–416.

Innovations in Hysteroscopy

Richa Sharma, Salvatore Giovanni Vitale, Gaetano Riemma, Rahul Manchanda

In last 30 years, many innovations in techniques and technologies have revolutionized the operative hysteroscopy. The French surgeon Antonin J. Desormeaux, in 1869, introduced the first functional endoscope and demonstrated, the first successful operative endoscopic procedures in living patients. In 1980, jacques Hamou introduced fine hysteroscopes of less than 5 mm, followed by Steffano Bettochi's atraumatic office hysteroscopes to "see and treat" in 1995. This ultimately revolutionized the field of Hysteroscopy. Technical innovations, simplified learning curve and the use of virtual reality training systems, have made hysteroscopic surgery accessible to younger gynecologists as well.

Modern innovations include ambulatory diagnostic and operative hysteroscopes for resectoscopy, ablation, cryoablation and morcellation.

Ambulatory services, has enabled us to perform diagnostic and operative hysteroscopy in an outpatient, office or in rural settings. This has provided much of the stimulus for the development of devices that will offer women a better hyste roscopy experience.

Advantages of Ambulatory Hysteroscopy

- It utilises a "one-stop" "see and treat" approach

- No need for cervical dilatation or any local anesthesia
- Avoid multiple patient visits through seamless consultation, testing, treatment or planning of clinical management
- Reduces hospital admissions
- Minimises the need to use expensive operation theater facilities.

This chapter discusses both diagnostic and operative hysteroscopic innovations.

Feasibility of ambulatory hysteroscopy depends upon the size of hysteroscope, because cervical dilatation is not needed if the diameter is less than 5 mm (Fig. 8.1).

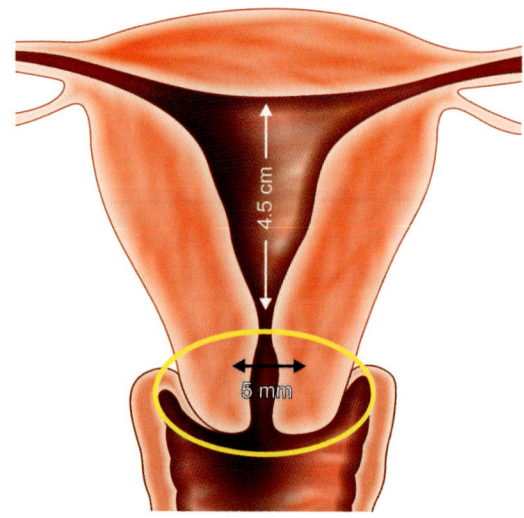

Fig. 8.1: Feasibility of ambulatory hysteroscopy—cervical canal diameter

Types of Innovations

1. **Ambulatory diagnostic hysteroscopy:** Endosee office hysteroscope
2. **Advanced miniaturized mechanical instruments**
   - Vitale biopsy snake" forceps
   - Intrauterine palpator
   - Accardi's microrotate instruments
3. **Mounir's modified inner sheath office**
4. **Mounir's pumpino**
5. **Ambulatory operative hysteroscopy**
   - *Office resectoscope*
     - 7 mm princess resectoscope
     - Accardi's 18.5 Fr hybrid Mono/Bipolar miniresectoscope
     - Gubbini mini hystero-resectoscope
     - Karl Storz® mini resectoscope
   - *Ambulatory ablation devices*
     - Minitouch ablation device
     - Minerva endometrial ablator
     - Cerene cryoablation device
     - Lina Librata
     - Mara water endometrial ablation device.

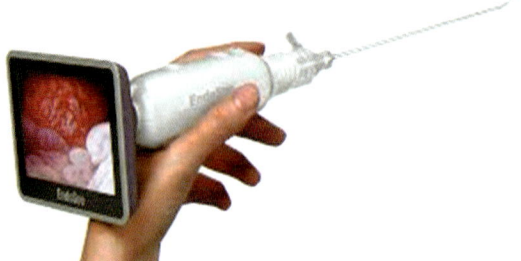

Fig. 8.2: EndoSee™ office hysteroscope

ADVANCED MINIATURIZED MECHANICAL INSTRUMENTS

Vitale Biopsy Snake Forceps

Biopsy snake forceps sec. VITALE (Centre lSRL, Ponte San Nicolò, Padua, Italy) is a unique-shaped forceps designed to be used with all 5 Fr hysteroscopes. These forceps are characterized by a sleeve with an opening along the whole width suited with a lancet with serrated edges fixed to one end, with a U-shaped joint and two sharp-edged spoon tongs that completely retract the lancet when clenched (Fig. 8.3).

Once the endometrial area to be inspected has been focused, the biopsy can be performed introducing the forceps through

ENDOSEE™ OFFICE HYSTEROSCOPE
(EndoSee Corp. Los Altos, California, United States)

It is a handheld, battery-operated, readily portable system with minimal setup (Fig. 8.2).

Parts

- Hand Tower™—incorporating a rechargeable battery lasts more than 2 hours
- Video and control electronics
- Touch screen 3.5 inch LCD display
- Sterile, disposable flexible hysteroscopic cannula of size less than 5 mm with a camera and light source at the tip
- Fluid distension medium is delivered via 30 inch intravenous standard bore extension tubing connected to cannula.

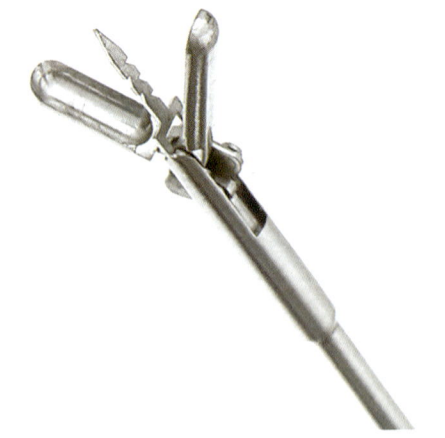

Fig. 8.3: The snake Vitale forceps. Focus on the lancet between the clamps

the hysteroscope. The opening of the clamps will push forward the lancet which will easily resect the tissue as necessary, through a simple traction motion, and using the anchoring action of the serrated edges.

Intrauterine Palpator

The Karl Storz® graduate intrauterine palpator (Karl Storz SE and Co.KG, Tuttlingen, Germany) is specifically designed to improve the precision of hysteroscopic metroplasty. With this 5 Fr instrument, it is possible to measure the length of the uterine cavity, together with the length of the cervix, and the resected septum. It is a reusable and robust instrument which is compatible for the operative channel of all modern miniaturized hysteroscopes (Fig. 8.4).

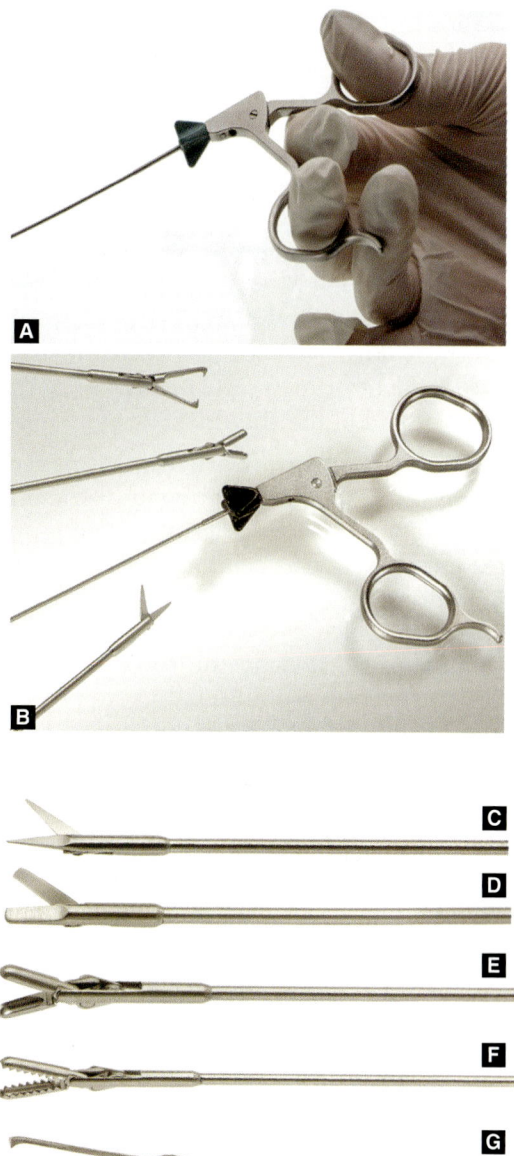

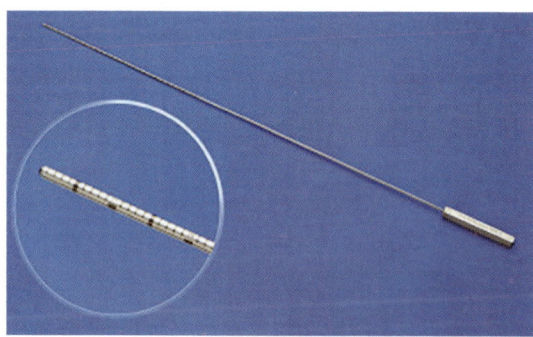

Fig. 8.4: The graduate intrauterine palpator

Accardi's Microrotate Instruments

RZ-Medizintechnik, Tuttlingen, Germany)

These are rotating hysteroscopic mechanical 5 Fr instruments, that have 360° rotation of the forceps with finger, avoiding the unnatural movement of the wrist, elbow and shoulder. The advantage of forceps rotational movement which results in a screwing on the base of the polyp including larger-based polyps, avoiding scissors usage and thus saves time. The same concept is applied to endometrial biopsy, with the continuous rotation to the classic "grasping biopsy", it reaches uterine wall areas that are more difficult to reach (Fig. 8.5A to G).

Fig. 8.5A to G: Accardi's microrotate instruments

About the Office Instruments

- Instruments are 25% lighter than other instruments.
- Lotus effect of the instruments iron, treatment of the surface to make water slide better on the surface.
- *Autoblocking system*: Due to the autoblocking system mechanism, the branches

of the forceps remain automatically closed and locked, no need to exert any force to the handle, keeping the tissue fragment locked inside the branches and allowing the operator to free the operating hand.

- *Rotating system*: The rotation of the instrument on its major axis, due to the simple wheel positioned between the handle and the stem, that allows the 360° rotation of the forceps with a simple finger. Thus avoiding the unnatural rotation of the wrist, elbow and the movement of the shoulder.

The use of rotation during biopsy or polypectomy adds the rotating movement to the right or left on the fulcrum of the tissue area to be removed, facilitating its removal. The continuous rotation movement is useful in polypectomies, as the continuous rotation mechanism exerted by the forceps on the base of the polyp, can easily remove the pathology without use the scissors. Thus the need to change the instruments during the procedure is avoided.

MOUNIR'S PUMPINO—NOVAL OFFICE HYSTEROMET

Pumpino is an office friendly, low budget, tight space designed hysteromet. The simple control with color screen, makes hysteroscopy a single operator procedure. This saves a lot of time and mess. The new design ensures the simplicity of direct flow rate control by putting the default option of a big rotary knob. Precise usage of this option, not only enhances an optional visual experience but also results in a decreased fluid usage (Fig. 8.6).

MOUNIR'S MODIFIED INNER SHEATH OFFICE (MIS-O)

Introduction of inner sheath alone in office hysteroscopy is more difficult than combined introduction of inner and outer sheaths, due to following reasons:

- It prevents smooth insertion of hysteroscope by trapping tissues in working channel.
- Leads to frequent blockage of working channel that causes, it an inconvenient procedure.
- It leaves distal tip unprotected and un-covered.

Features of MIS-O (Fig. 8.7)

- Sheath is elongated up to the length of telescope
- Matting distal 3 mm into single cavity (pressure room)
- Trimming inner sheath tip to align with 30° lens tip
- Smoothing of tip edges

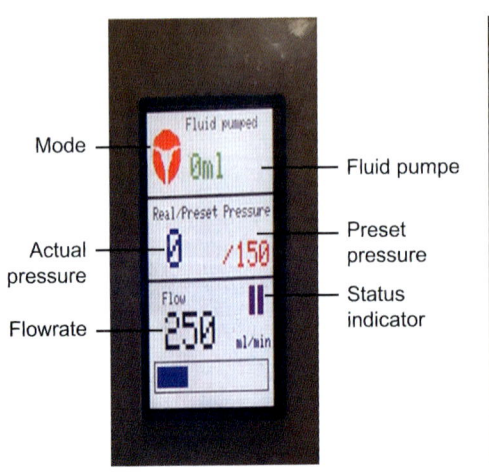

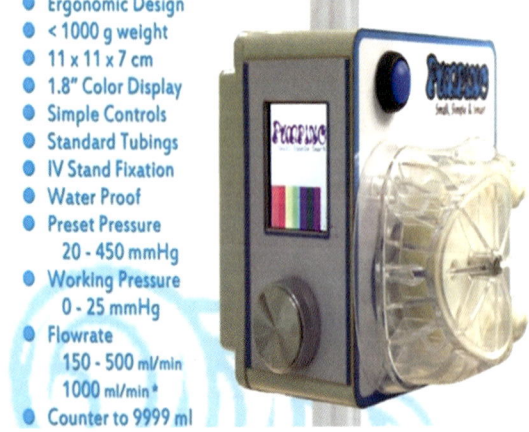

- Ergonomic Design
- < 1000 g weight
- 11 x 11 x 7 cm
- 1.8" Color Display
- Simple Controls
- Standard Tubings
- IV Stand Fixation
- Water Proof
- Preset Pressure
  20 - 450 mmHg
- Working Pressure
  0 - 25 mmHg
- Flowrate
  150 - 500 ml/min
  1000 ml/min*
- Counter to 9999 ml

Fig. 8.6: Mounir's pumpino—office hysteromet

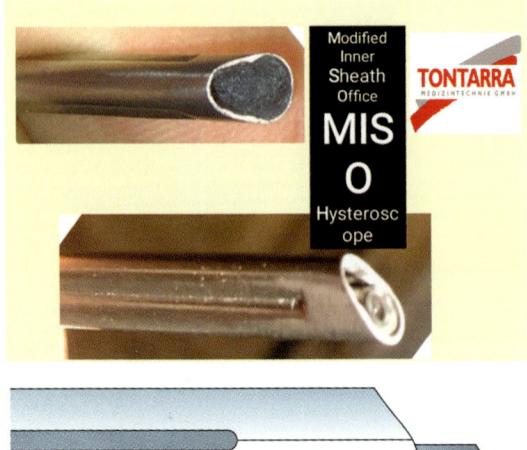

Fig. 8.7: Mounir's modified inner sheath office

Advantages

- Double diameter cost effective hysteroscopes.
- No need to buy a separate diagnostic sheath.
- Using oval tip instead of circular tip of diameter, provides atraumatic and easy insertion.

7 MM PRINCESS RESECTOSCOPE

The Princess resectoscope (Richard Wolf GmbH, Knittlingen, Germany) ensures minimal dilation and trauma to the cervical canal due to its 7 mm diameter, helping to challenge also the stenotic canal (Fig. 8.8).

Nonetheless, a strength is the freedom of movement which is made possible by means of a two-rotating-sheath system. This allows the working part of the resectoscope to rotate through 360° in the absence of a rotation of the outer sheath inside the cervical channel.

The instrument works both with mono or bipolar current. Especially, the bipolar vaporization electrode "BIVAP" (Richard Wolf GmbH, Knittlingen, Germany) can be used with clear results to perform endometrial ablation and myomas resection with or without pharmacological preparation of the endometrium.

ACCARDI'S 18.5 Fr HYBRID MONO/ BIPOLAR MINI-RESECTOSCOPE
Grazia mini-resectoscope, RZ Medizintechnik, Tuttlingen, Germany

This mini-resectoscope 18.5 Fr. has been introduced, which being "halfway" between 15 Fr. and 26 Fr. promises to be an excellent compromise between the two well-established instruments. It is made of titanium, equipped with a rotating mechanism, equipped with cutting loop and cold knife with a size of about 6 mm and various shapes, from the most classic (Loop 90°) to some with original shape; considering the electrosurgical point of view the instrument is hybrid and can use both monopolar and bipolar energy. With regard to the optics it is possible to use the classic 2.9 mm, 30° or 0° degrees optics (Fig. 8.9).

Advantages

- Can perform vaginoscopy, direct uterine access without cervical dilatation.
- Effective for uterine septa, endometrial ablation, endometrial and cervical polyps, myoma G0/G1/G2, isthmocele or any other uterine pathology.
- 6 mm loop of 18.5 Fr with "tear-loop" of 16 Fr resectoscope, guarantees a major cutting edge allowing faster surgery.

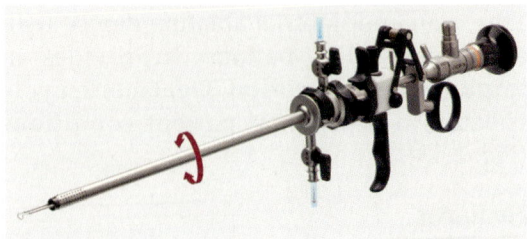

Fig. 8.8: Princess™ resectoscope

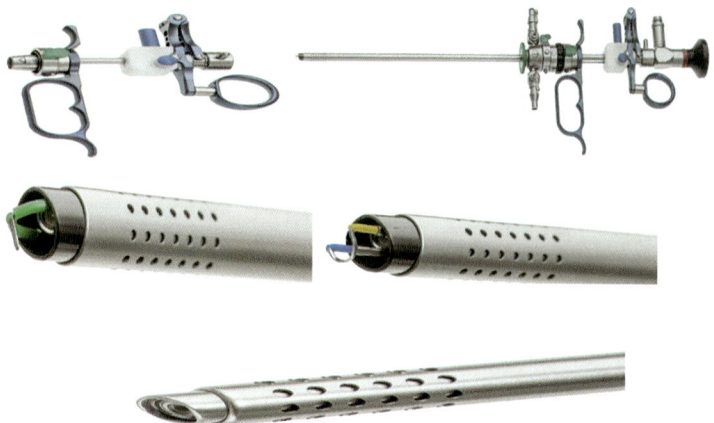

Fig. 8.9: Accardi's 18.5 Fr hybrid mono/bipolar mini-resectoscope

KARL STORZ® MINI/RESECTOSCOPE

A 15 Fr resectoscope designed by Karl Storz® (Karl Storz SE and Co.KG, Tuttlingen, Germany). This bipolar instrument allows to perform resection of polyps, small sub-mucous fibroids, septa, synechiae and other intrauterine pathologies in an ambulatory setting. Due to its small diameter, it requires no anesthesia and with little or even no dilation of the cervix (Fig. 8.10).

It has been developed to be used with an Autocon® III 400 HF generator (Karl Storz SE and Co.KG, Tuttlingen, Germany) in order to guarantee successful resection, together with coagulation and vaporization. This 16 Fr mini-resectoscope can be switched into a diagnostic device by means of semirigid mechanical instruments such as

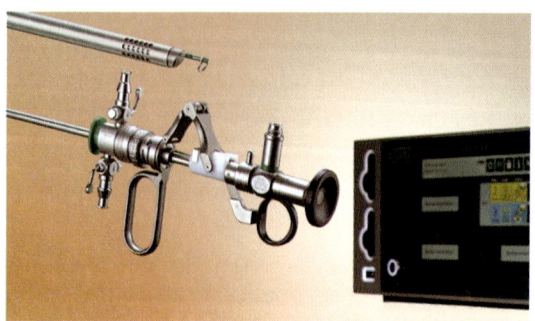

Fig. 8.10: Karl Storz® 16 Fr mini-resectoscope

grasp forceps or blunt scissors. The formation of plasma allows the mini-resectoscope to produce self-cleaning loops which enhance the operator's vision.

MINITOUCH ENDOMETRIAL ABLATOR

(Minitouch, Ltd., MicroCube, LLC)

It is an office endometrial ablator used for a novel thermal endometrial ablation technique. It has flexibile 3.5 mm diameter and delivers microwave energy via induction loop (Fig. 8.11 A to C). Ablation is simple and done in 60 seconds (Fig. 8.12). The main advantage is that there is no need to time the procedure, it can be performed any time before, during, or after the periods.

MINERVA ENDOMETRIAL ABLATION SYSTEM

(Minerva Surgical Inc., Redwood City, CA, USA, FDA approved in July 2015

This is an endometrial ablation device with a cervical sealing balloon. It provides an impedance controlled treatment cycle specific to individual patient conditions (Fig. 8.13).

Features

- Fast procedure time 3 to 4 minutes (device insertion to device removal).

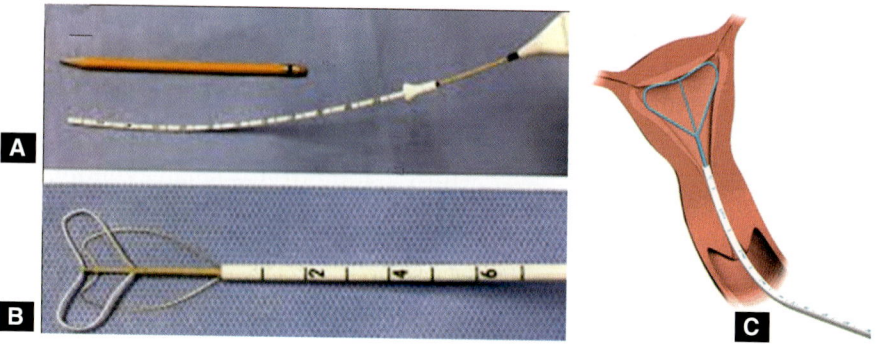

Fig. 8.11A to C: Minitouch endometrial ablator

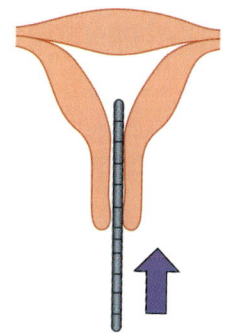
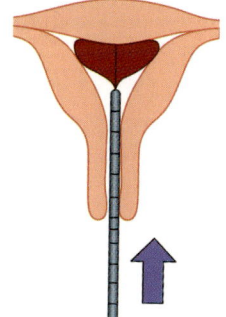
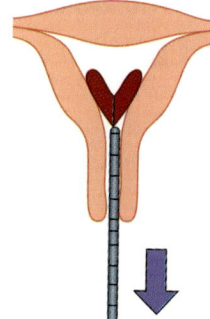

The flexible minitouch device is gently introduce into the uterus

Soft end of the device opens and conforms to the uterus. A gently warming 2–3 minute treatment cycle is initiated

Treatment automatically stops when completed, and the device is gently removed

Fig. 8.12: Working principle

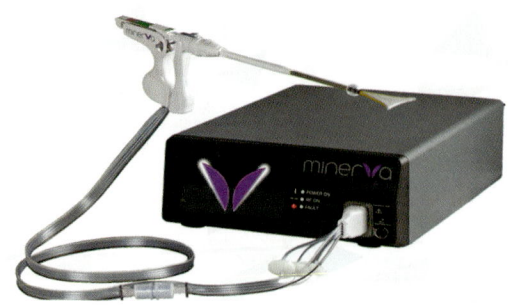

Fig. 8.13: Minerva endometrial ablation system

- Silicone membrane array-lubricious nature of silicone facilitates easy insertion, sealing, and a non-stick atraumatic removal.
- Patented uterine integrity test (UIT)—automatically checks the integrity of the uterine cavity.

- Cervical sealing balloon—seals the cervical canal near the internal os.
- No measurement entry needed—No uterine length/width controller entries are required
- Low power delivered—40 watts

Working of Minerva

Involves the combination of 3 mechanisms of ablation that creates a uniform and reproducible ablation of the endometrium.

1. Hot Array Membrane

Plasma releases thermal energy in the form of heat which ablates surrounding endometrial tissue that is in direct contact with the silicone array membrane (Fig. 8.14A).

2. Heated Intra-cavitary Fluids

Hot retained cavity fluids heated by the membrane ablate tissue not in direct contact with the silicone array membrane (Fig. 8.14B).

3. RF Energy

Endometrial tissue is ablated with penetrating bipolar RF electrical current which also creates plasma by ionising argon (AR) gas that is fully contained in the silicone array membrane (Fig. 8.14C).

CERENE CRYOTHERAPY DEVICE

Channel Medsystems, Emeryville, CA-FDA approved in March 28, 2019 (Fig. 8.15A and B) It is an office endometrial cryoablation device, which uses cryothermic energy by

liquid-to-gas phase change of nitrous oxide to achieve ablation throughout the uterine cavity. Treatment cycle takes 2½ minutes.

Working Principle: Liquid nitrous oxide (originating from a small cylinder located in the device handle) flows through a delivery line and into an inflow line with multiple jets. Liquid N_2O is infused into an ultra-thin polyurethane liner, where it converts into gas. Gaseous N_2O is exhausted through the exhaust hose exiting the bottom of the handle. Exhaust collection, which connects to the exhaust hose exiting the bottom of the device.

Pre-requisites

- Refractory heavy menstrual bleeding with no definable organic cause.

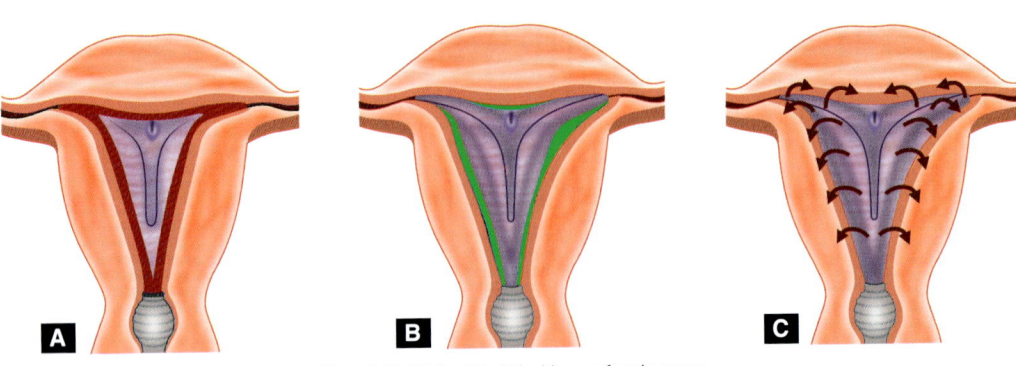

Fig. 8.14A to C: Working of minerva

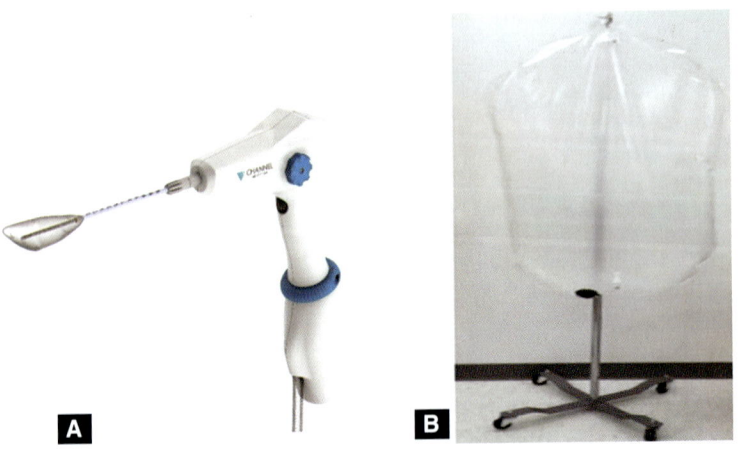

Fig. 8.15A and B: Cerene cryotherapy device

- Age 25 to 50 years
- Endometrial cavity measurements within the following parameters:
  a. Sounded length of uterine cavity (exocervix to fundus) no greater than 10 cm.
  b. Endometrial cavity length (internal os to fundus) must be between 2.5 and 6.5 cm.
  c. Myometrial thickness of at least 10 mm.

LINA LIBRATA

(LiNA Medical ApS, Denmark)

It is the first cordless fully automated, disposable Balloon ablation device that is ready out of the box. Simply insert the battery and press the 'ON' button to begin the pre-heating process It has 5.4 mm catheter requires minimal or no dilation and capable of treating irregular shaped uteri. It takes 2 minute duration for treatment time (Fig. 8.16).

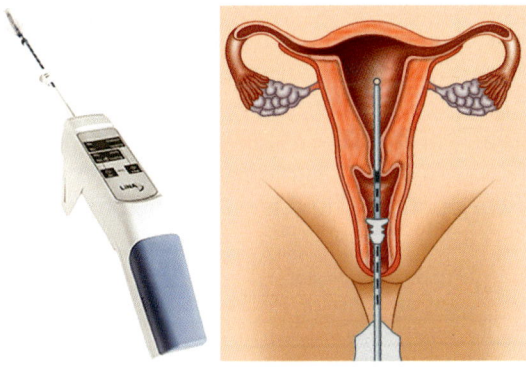

Fig. 8.16: Lina librata

Advantages

- Ideally suited Cordless Intelligence requiring, no generator or cables.
- Librata's intelligent software automatically manages time, temperature, and pressure for effective treatment.
- Continuous monitoring of uterine cavity for optimal safety.

MARA WATER VAPOR ABLATION TREATMENT SYSTEM

AEGEA Medical, Menlo Park California, FDA-approved in June 2017

It has patented Smart Seal™ and Integrity Pro™ technology (Fig. 8.17).

It is an office ablation procedure with no requirement of dilatation or anesthesia.

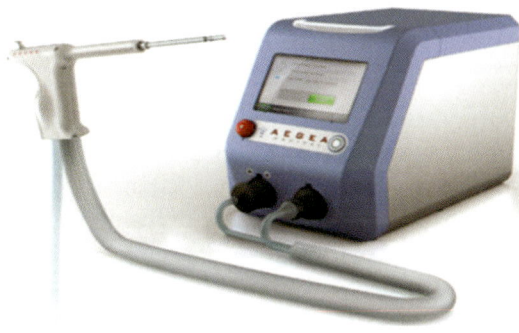

Fig. 8.17: Mara Water Vapor Ablation treatment system

Advantages

Ablation can be done in following situations:
- Uterine cavities up to 12 cm in length
- Any uterine width
- Uterine cavities with certain types of fibroids
- Patients with a prior LSCS
- In the presence of essure

Working Occurs in Four Steps

1st step: Soft tip of the Mara Vapor Probe is gently inserted into the uterus (Fig. 8.18A).

2nd step: 3 balloons automatically inflate to seal the uterus and secure the probe. Uterine cavity safety tests are completed before water vapor treatment begins (Fig. 8.18B).

3rd step: Delivery of water vapor is carefully controlled to treat the endometrial lining and total duration is 2 minutes. At the end of the procedure, the balloons automatically deflate, and the Vapor Probe is removed (Fig. 8.18C).

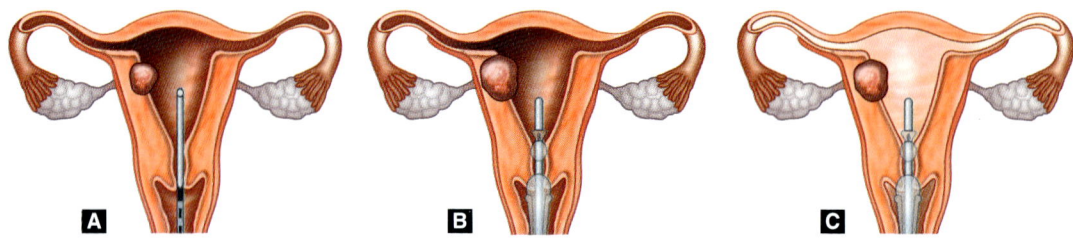

Fig. 18.18A to C: Working principle

GUBBINI MINI-HYSTERO-RESECTOSCOPES

Tontarra Medizintechnik GmbH, Wurmlingen, Germany

Optimization of "see and treat" approach by simply exchanging the diagnostic working sheath with the inner continous flow resectoscopic sheath—without the need of re-introduction of the outer sheath. Main advantage is that the diagnostic and operative resectoscopy can be performed in one session (Fig. 8.19).

Advantages

a. Office resectoscopy can be done without the need for:
- Vaginal instruments (speculum, dilators, tenaculum, etc.)
- Cervical dilatation and efficient in stenotic os
- Anesthesia or analgesia

b. Even 90° resections possible

c. Short operating time

d. Bipolar current mode increases safety

TruClear Hysteroscopic Tissue Removal System (Fig. 8.20)

8.0 and 5C (Medtronic, Minneapolis, Minnesota), FDA approved 2005 1st Generation hystero-scopic morcellator that work with physiologic saline solution as distension and irrigation media. It does not use high frequency electric current but a mechanical approach to remove intrauterine tissue. For this reason, there is no damage coming from thermal energy or energy discharge. Nonetheless, no bubbles or electrical energy in the uterus reduces the risk of air or gas emboli and the risk of patient harm. The system is made of the control unit, handpiece, and foot switch. The usage of TruClear® guarantees the minimization of tissue floating inside the uterine cavity. A clear operative field is maintained by means

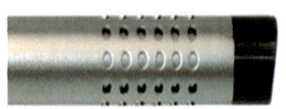

Round tip with small diameter: 16 Fr

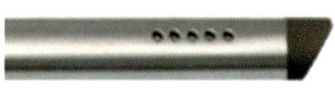

Elliptic formed tip for an easier introduction into the cervical canal. Average diameter: 14,9 Fr, ~15 Fr

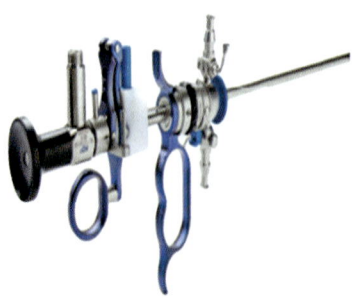

Fig. 8.19: Gubbini mini-hystero-resectoscopes

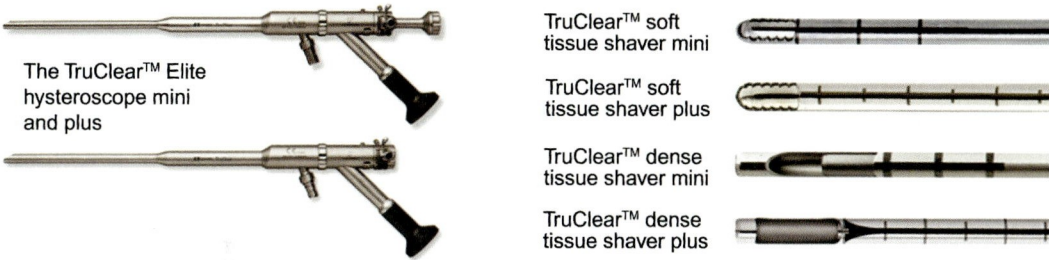

Fig. 8.20: Truclear hysteroscopic tissue removal system

of a continuous flow and suction system. A strength of this instrument is that it provides fewer procedural steps due to a single insertion program, becoming an easy-to-use device.

TruClear 8.0–8 mm diameter with a 9 mm rigid sheath.

TruClear 5C hysteroscopy system incorporates a 2.9 mm rotatory-style blade through a 5 mm, 0° hysteroscope.

Functioning of TruClear

Figure 8.21A to E shows functioning of TruClear.

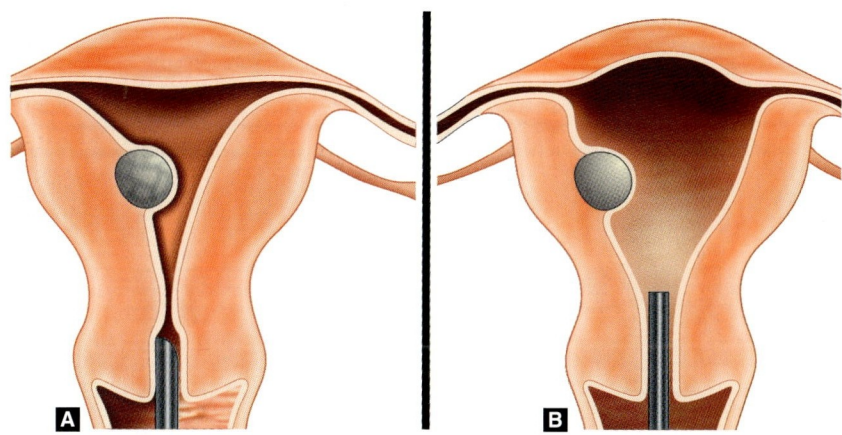

Fig. 8.21A and B: Functioning of TruClear: (A) Insert the truClear into the cavity; (B) distend the cavity with saline

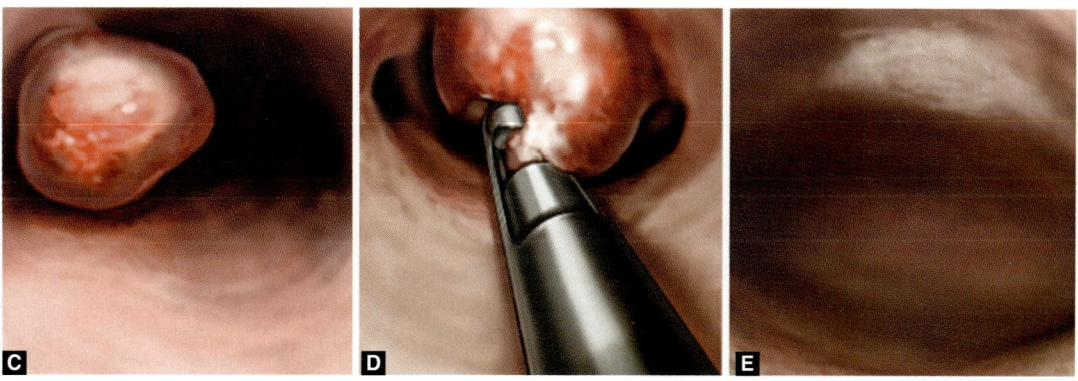

Fig. 8.21C to E: TruClear hysteroscopy working. Locate the intrauterine pathology—truClear will simultaneously cut and aspirate

Table 8.1: Types of MyoSure Devices (Fig. 8.22)				
MyoSure devices	*Myosure LITE*	*MyoSure*	*MyoSure REACH*	*MyoSure XL*
Tissue recommended	Polyps <3 cm	All polyps Fibroids <3 cm	All polyps Fibroids <3 cm	All intrauterine pathology
Device outer diameter	3 mm	3 mm	3 mm	4 mm
Duration	3 cm polyp in 2 min	3 cm fibroid in 10 min	3 cm fibroid in 10 min	5 cm fibroid in 15 min
Tissue removal rate	7 gm/min (polyp tissue)	1.5 gm/min (fibroid tissue)	1.5 gm/min (fibroid tissue)	4.3 gm/min (fibroid tissue)

MYOSURE TISSUE REMOVAL SYSTEM

(Hologic, Bedford, MA) FDA approved in 2009

It is a 2nd generation hysteroscopic morcella-tor and helpful for OPD basis removal of polyps, fibroids, intrauterine pathologies (Fig. 8.22). No analgesia or local anesthesia is needed.

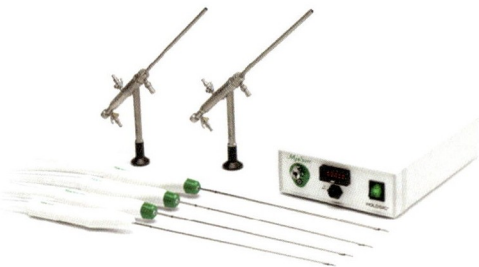

Fig. 8.22: MyoSure tissue removal system

✍ Key points

1. Ambulatory services, has enabled us to perform diagnostic and operative hysteroscopy in an outpatient, office or in rural settings.
2. Modern innovations includes ambulatory diagnostic and operative hysteroscopes for resectoscopy, ablation, cryoablation and Morcellation.
3. Feasibility of Ambulatory Hysteroscopy depends upon the size of hysteroscope, because cervical dilatation is not needed if the diameter is less than 5 mm.
4. Mounir's pumpino is a novel office friendly, low budget, tight space designed hysteromat.

5. Accardi's microrotate instruments are rotating Hysteroscopic mechanical 5 Fr instruments, that has 360 degree rotation of the forceps with finger, avoiding the unnatural movement of the wrist, elbow and shoulder.
6. Vitale biopsy snake" forceps is specially designed instrument, opening of the clamps will push forward the lancet which will easily resect the tissue as necessary, through a simple traction motion, and using the anchoring action of the serrated edges.
7. Accardi's 18.5 Fr hybrid mini-resectoscope can be used with both monopolar and bipolar energy.

BIBLIOGRAPHY

1. Amer-Cuenca JJ, Marín-Buck A, Vitale SG, La Rosa VL, Caruso S, Cianci A, Lisón JF. Non-pharmacological pain control in outpatient hysteroscopies. Minim Invasive Ther Allied Technol. 2019 Feb 22:1–10. doi: 10.1080/13645706.2019.1576054.

2. Casadio P, Gubbini G, Morra C, Franchini M, Paradisi R, Seracchioli R. Channel-like 360° Isthmocele Treatment with a 16F Mini-Resecto-scope: A Step-by-step Technique. J Minim Invasive Gynecol. 2019 May 3. pii: S1553–4650(19)30212-2. doi: 10.1016/j.jmig.2019.04.024.

3. Dealberti D, Riboni F, Cosma S, Pisani C, Montella F, Saitta S, Calagna G, Di SpiezioSardo A. Feasibility and Acceptability of Office-Based Polypectomy With a 16F Mini-Resectoscope: A Multicenter Clinical Study. J Minim Invasive Gynecol. 2016 Mar-Apr;23(3):418–24. doi: 10.1016/j.jmig.2015.12.016.

4. Di Tommaso S, Cavallotti C, Malvasi A, Vergara D, Rizzello A, De Nuccio F, Tinelli A. A Qualitative and Quantitative Study of the Innervation of the Human Non-Pregnant Uterus.Curr Protein Pept Sci. 2017;18(2):140–148. doi: 10.2174/1389203717666160330105341.

5. Franchini M, Lippi G, Calzolari S, Giarrè G, Gubbini G, Catena U, Di SpiezioSardo A, Florio P. Hysteroscopic Endometrial Polypectomy: Clinical and Economic Data in Decision Making. J Minim Invasive Gynecol. 2018 Mar-Apr;25(3): 418–425. doi: 10.1016/j.jmig.2017.08.001.

6. Noventa M, Ancona E, Quaranta M, Vitagliano A, Cosmi E, D'Antona D, Gizzo S. Intrauterine Morcellator Devices: The Icon of Hysteroscopic Future or Merely a Marketing Image? A Systematic Review Regarding Safety, Efficacy, Advantages, and Contraindications. Reprod Sci. 2015 Oct; 22(10):1289–96. doi: 10.1177/1933719115578929.

7. Papalampros P, Gambadauro P, Papadopoulos N, Polyzos D, Chapman L, Magos A. The mini-resectoscope: a new instrument for office hysteroscopic surgery. ActaObstetGynecol Scand. 2009;88(2):227–30. doi: 10.1080/00016340802516585.

8. Salazar, CA, and Isaacson, K B (2018). Office Operative Hysteroscopy: An Update. Journal of Minimally Invasive Gynecology, 25(2), 199—208. doi:10.1016/j.jmig.2017.08—009.

9. Vitale SG, Caruso S, Vitagliano A, Vilos G, Di Gregorio LM, Zizolfi B, Tesarik J, Cianci A. The value of virtual reality simulators in hysteroscopy and training capacity: a systematic review. Minim Invasive Ther Allied Technol. 2019 Jun 6:1–9. doi: 10.1080/13645706.2019. 1625404. [Epub ahead of print] PubMed PMID: 31169414.

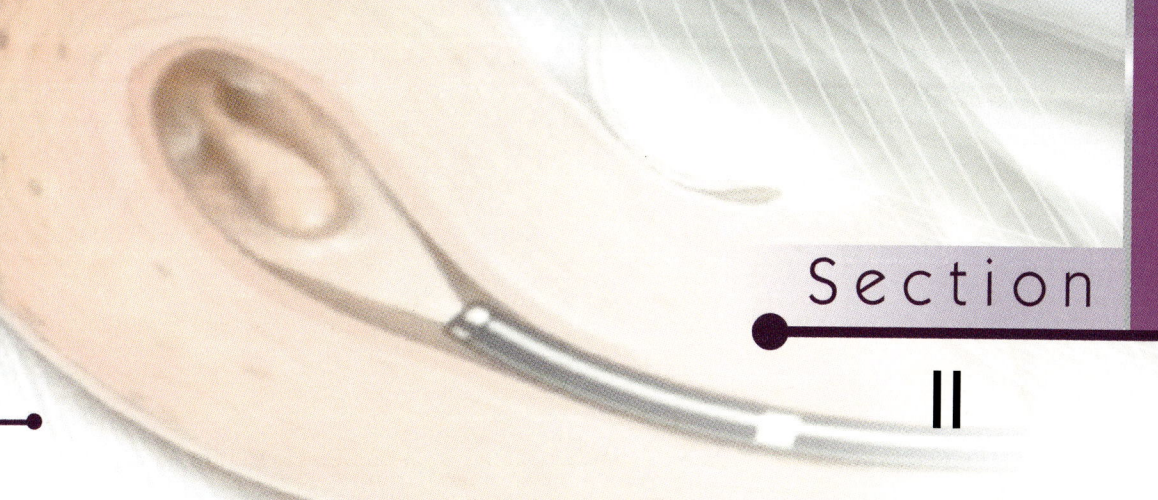

Different Case Scenarios

Management Algorithms: Diagnosis, Appropriate Preoperative Preparations and Postoperative Management

- Case 1: Cervical Stenosis
- Case 2: Hemorrhage
- Case 3: Uterine Perforation
- Case 4: Saline Media induced Operative Hysteroscopy Intravascular Absorption (OHIA) Syndrome or Glycine Media induced Gynecological TURP Syndrome
- Case 5: Air Embolism

Cervical Stenosis

Mario Franchini, Giampietro Gubbini, Richa Sharma, Rahul Manchanda

A 28-year-old woman with primary infertility, was anxious to conceive. Her Gynecologist failed to perform the office hysteroscopy at first attempt and on second attempt false passage was created.
Diagnosis—Cervical Stenosis

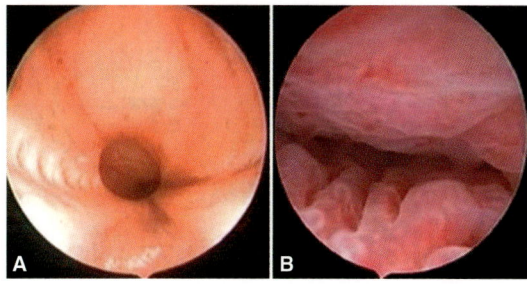

Fig. 1A and B: External cervical ostium nulliparous, multiparous

INTRODUCTION

Cervical stenosis is a challenging clinical entity that requires prompt identification and management in order to avoid iatrogenic injury at the time of endocervical canal cannulation. Extreme uterine retroversion or anteversion and cervical stenosis may limit the ability to introduce the hysteroscope and there is a risk of creation of a false passage or perforation. Thus care should be taken, while using an appropriate technique.

Clinical bimanual examination and ultrasound evaluation may help to identify these anatomical modifications. Since almost half of the complications at hysteroscopy are related to cervical entry, caution should be employed at this stage of the procedure. Nevertheless, most cases of cervical stenosis are solved by using the distal oval tip of the hysteroscope to separate the fibers.

"Cervix" is a term derived from the Latin word for "neck," denoting a constricted part of an organ. There are minimal data that describe the diameter, length of cervical canal and shape of the external cervical ostium (ECO) in healthy women or in women with reproductive tract diseases. The ECO is small and round in a nulliparous woman but appears as a larger transverse slit in a multiparous woman (Fig. 1A and B). The diameter of ECO in nulliparous women is in

the range of 5–8 mm. ECO stenosis has been defined, when the diameter is less than 4.5 mm and if there is difficult access that requires special maneuvers to introduce the hysteroscope into the cervical canal.

Patient selection is very important.

Cervical stenosis should be anticipated in the following

Various cervical stenosis sites (Fig. 2A to D)

i. Nulliparous
ii. Postmenopausal cervix
iii. Previous Cervical Procedures (cone biopsy, perforation, cervical laceration, curettage, cesarean section)

Bettocchi's Classification for Cervical Stenosis on the Basis of Localization of Stenosis

Type I—pin point
ICO type II—stenosis of distal third of cervical channel and the internal cervical ostium
Type III—stenosis of the ICO
Type IV—combined stenosis of ECO and ICO with or without anteflexed or retroflexed uterus.

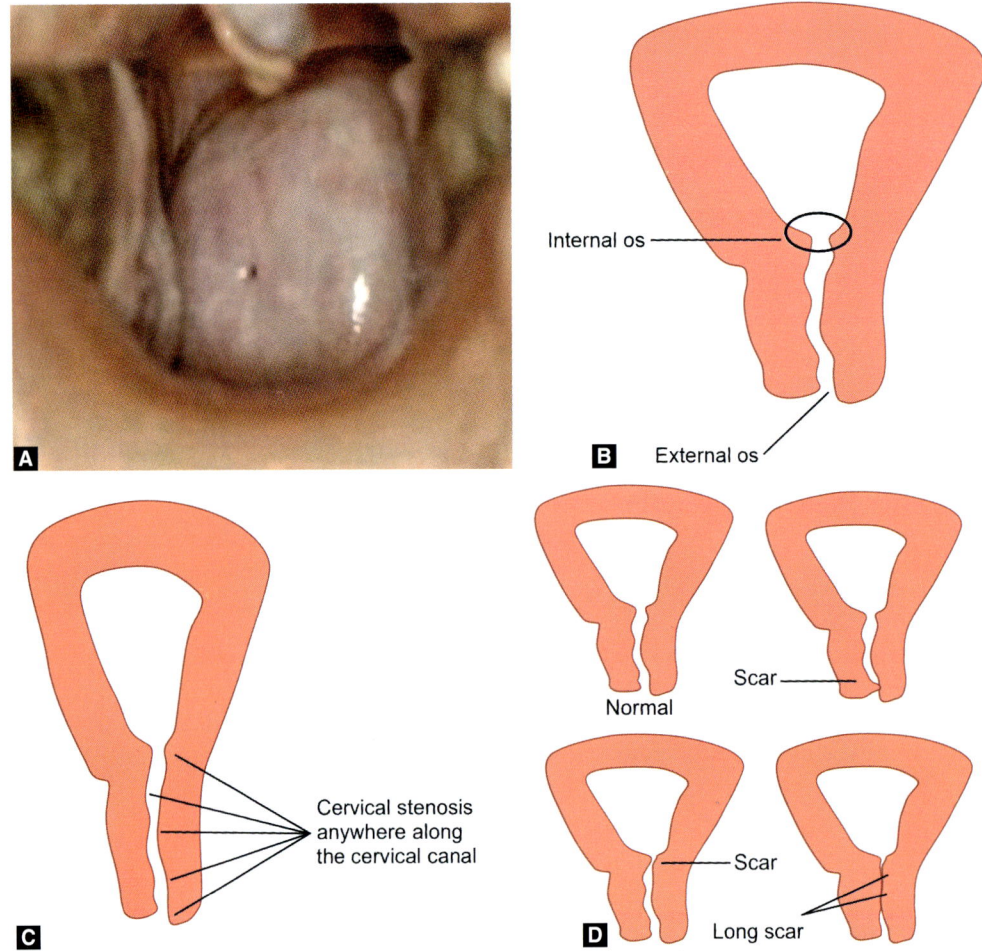

Fig. 2A to D: Cervical stenosis

Cervical Stenosis Classification based on Etiologies

Congenital or acquired

- **Congenital cervical stenosis** is observed as result of disorders of vertical fusion of the Müllerian ducts and is generally associated with uterine malformations and vaginal septum.
- **Acquired:** Scarring after previous surgical procedures (cone biopsy) on the lower part of cervix is the most common cause of acquired cervical stenosis. Furthermore, previous false passage, perforation, cervical laceration or cesarean section may be involved in cervical stenosis of the upper part of cervical canal.

Preoperative preparations: A stenotic cervix increases the difficulty of office hysteroscopic procedures. Preoperative cervical ripening minimises cervical complications and could be used in selected cases.

Preoperative cervical priming with following agents:

- Misoprostol (off label) 200–400 µg buccal/sublingual/intravaginal the night before hysteroscopy (ACOG 2018)
- Misoprostol 400 mg either orally or vaginally 6–8 h prior to surgery or 400 mg sublingually 2–4 hr prior to surgery.
- Hygroscopic dilators—lamineria tents or Dilapan: S (3 × 55 mm or 4 × 55 mm) 12 h before procedure.

- Intracervical injection of vasopressin solution (4 IU in 100 cc sodium chloride) injected at the 4 and 8 o'clock positions

Intraoperative Management

1. **Entry under direct vision with vaginoscopic approach and speculum assisted:** Historically the first diagnostic hysteroscopic procedures were performed placing a vaginal speculum and tenaculum to gain the visualization of the cervix using carbon dioxide as distension medium.

   In 1997, Bettocchi et al. developed the "vaginoscopic approach" or "no-touch technique" for the atraumatic insertion of the hysteroscope into ECO, without the aid of the speculum, the tenaculum and any local or general anesthesia. The scope is introduced directly into the posterior vaginal fornix and the vaginal vault is distended with saline. Pulling back a 30° rigid scope the ECO can be visualized. To avoid the vaginoscopic approach, speculum assisted hysteroscopy is an entry technique performed using the speculum without the tenaculum to gain the visualization of ECO. Speculum can be removed once, hysteroscope is inserted

The scope can then be guided and advanced gently along the axis of the cervical canal maintaining the scope located in the middle of the canal and rotating the entire scope from 6 o'clock to 3 or 9 o'clock. This approach reduces patient discomfort avoiding stimulation of the muscle fibers of cervical canal.

2. **Over passing cervical stenosis:** The access to the uterine cavity represents the main limiting factors to the widespread use of office hysteroscopy. Currently, a wide set of 5 Fr semirigid instruments, mechanical (scissors-graspers), electrical (monopolar or bipolar electrode) and laser probe, may be used to overcome stenosis of the cervical canal in an office setting. The instruments may be inserted in the operating channel of a rigid 5–4 mm hysteroscope and used to dilate or cut the fibrous tissue responsible for the stenosis under direct visualization (Flowchart 1).

Cervical Stenosis with Light Fibrosis

Optical rotation technique: Pin point ECO with light fibrosis, may be dilated with the distal oval tip of the hysteroscope. Rigid scopes have a bevel tip, which gives the

Flowchart 1: Management algorithm

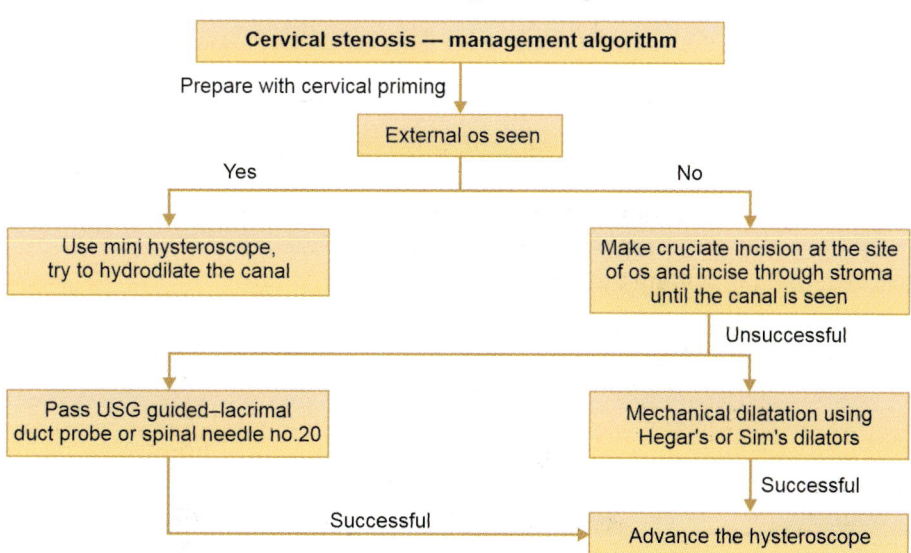

capacity for tissue penetration and ability to separate the fibers. Most cases of cervical stenosis are resolved by rotating the scope on the camera.

Mechanical entry: Alternatively, the light fibrosis can be stretched by grasping forceps inserted within ECO with the jaws closed and then gently opened to dilate the cervix just enough to introduce the tip of the hysteroscope (Fig. 3).

Cervical Stenosis with Dense Fibrosis

Entrance with sharp scissors or bipolar/monopolar electrode: When a dense fibrosis is present, the fibrous ring may be cut using sharp scissors (Fig. 4A) or bipolar/

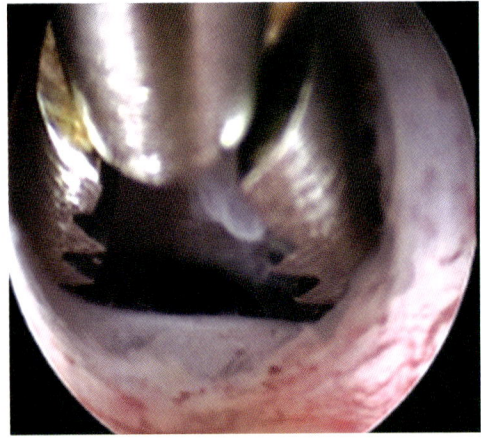

Fig. 3: Cervical stenosis opening with grasper

monopolar electrode (Fig. 4B), creating three or four radial incisions, at approximately the 3, 6, 9 and 12 o'clock positions extending ECO and allowing the passage of the hysteroscope. Sometimes the use of scissors is needed to cut the lateral corner of the cervical canal or fibrous tissue adhesions at the level of the internal os.

Generally, the most used strategy to overpass all types of ECO and cervical canal stenosis is to perform a cold adhesiolysis with the distal tip of a scope in combination with miniaturized instruments. Finally, hydrodilation may be helpful to advance minimizing trauma to the cervical canal. There is evidence describing that the injection of a dilute solution of vasopressin (0.05 U/mL) at the cervical stroma, significantly reduces the force needed to dilate the cervix. This technique could be an alternative when faced with a stenotic cervix in a patient who has not received pre-procedure prostaglandin to prime the cervix (Flowchart 2).

Cervical disintegration: Cervical disintegration often occurs in patients with a history of invasive surgical procedures on the cervix such as traquelectomy or cold knife conization. In these cases, it is impossible to determine where the external os is located. The use of a miniaturized 5 Fr mechanical or

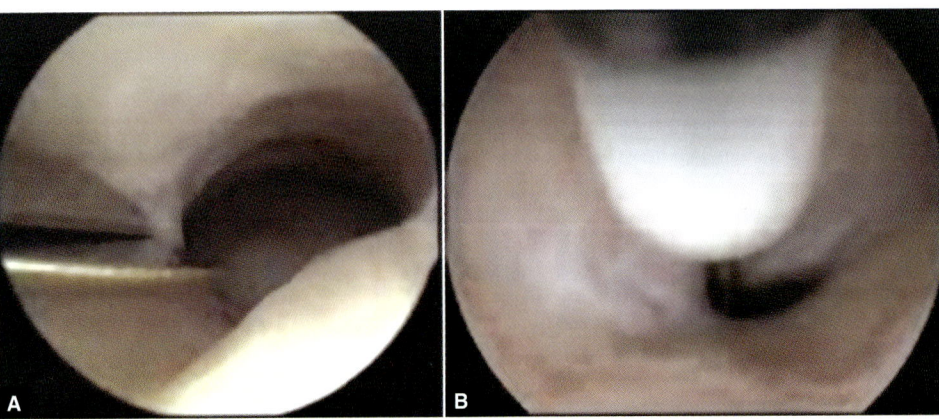

Fig. 4A and B: Cervical stenosis—cutting with scissors and electrode

Flowchart 2: Summary of management

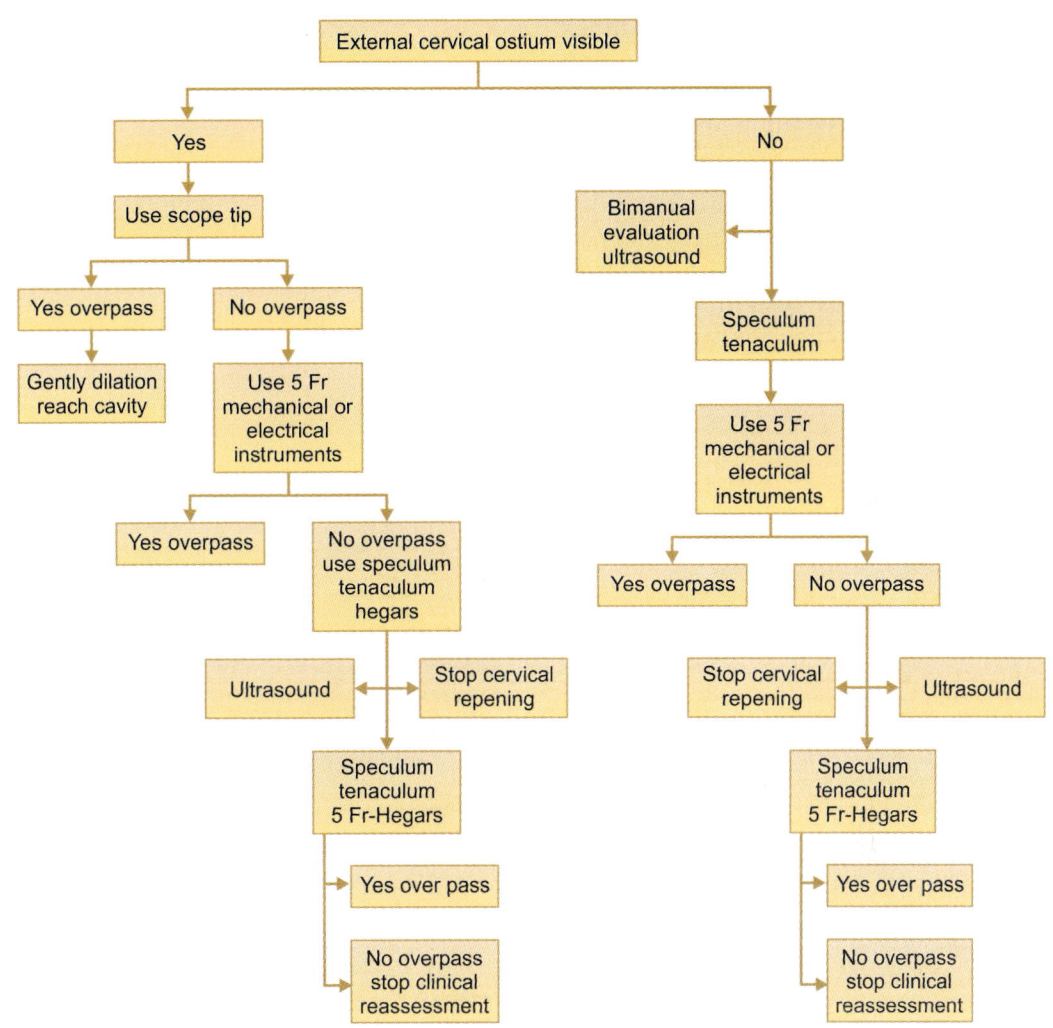

electrical instrumentation under hysteroscopic control and ultrasound guide often allows access to the unstructured cervix.

Another main reason for failed hysteroscopy is uterine malposition: Since malposition may increase the risk of uterine perforation and false passage during insertion of the hysteroscope, a clinical bimanual examination and ultrasound evaluation may help to identify these anatomical modifications.

Bimanual examination of an anteverted uterus combined with a severe degree of retroflexion (body of uterus is at 120° axis to anteverted axis of cervix) or a retroverted uterus combined with severe anteflexion (Figs 5 and 6) can lead to problems with hysteroscopic insertion and progression within the cervical canal. Failure of procedure, false passage and perforation may occur at the site of angle between the canal axis and body axis due to an apparent obstruction. Transvaginal ultrasound performed immediately before the procedure shows the body of uterus at 120° axis to anteverted axis of cervix with an acute angulation.

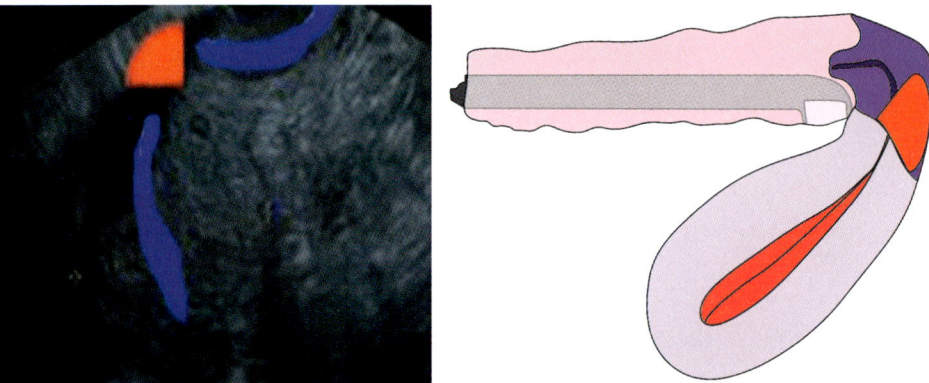

Fig. 5. Anteverted uterus combined with a severe degree of retroflexion. Ultrasound image shows body of uterus is at 120° axis to anteverted axis of cervix with acute angulation (red mark critical area for false passage or perforation)

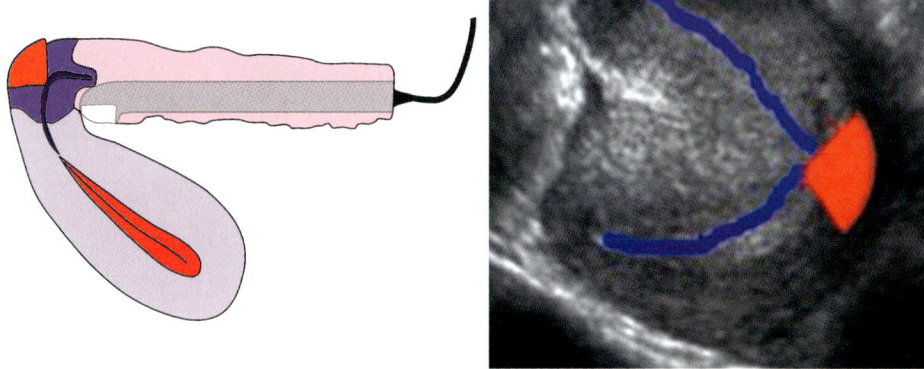

Fig. 6: Retroverted uterus combined with a severe degree of anteflexion. Ultrasound image shows body of uterus is at 120° axis to retroverted axis of cervix with acute angulation (red mark critical area for false passage or perforation)

The natural position of the uterus is classified by whether the ECO points are superiorly toward the bladder (retroversion), posteriorly toward the rectum (anteversion), or toward the introitus (axial position). Sonography is a useful and reliable method for determining the uterine axis and the angle between cervical canal (CC) and corpus. The fundus is usually further flexed in the direction dictated by the cervix, that is, anteverted and anteflexed or retroverted and retroflexed.

Management of Malpositioned Uterus

- **Acutely anteflexed uterus:** Place a long-bladed, open-sided Graves speculum deep in the anterior or posterior fornix, it pushes the fundus to the midposition and can facilitate dilation. Speculum can be removed once, hysteroscope is inserted.
- **Acutely retroflexed uterus:** Place a tenaculum on the posterior lip of the cervix and apply traction, it straightens the cervical canal.

Since pain is the primary reason for failure to complete hysteroscopy procedures in an outpatient setting, awareness of strategies for pain relief is generally considered critical. In our practice, we avoid any of the many available methods for achieving pain relief during office procedures for ECO stenosis, because the main advantage of hysteroscopy with vaginoscopic approach is the prompt identification of false passages and perforation. Therefore, a sudden increase of patient's pain and discomfort, bleeding, or the visualization of white/red tissue are warning signs of a false passage into the cervical fibro-myometrial tissue.

Management of Complications

Overcoming cervical stenosis is challenging and increases the risk of false passage and perforation.

Usually, a false passage or perforation may occur at the site of angle between the canal axis and body axis on the anterior wall in an anteverted uterus combined with a severe degree of retroflexion and in posterior wall in a retroverted uterus combined with a severe degree of anteflexion. Therefore, the risk of damage of cervical vessels is unlikely to occur in these sites and the risk of bleeding is minimum using mechanical dissection (Fig. 7).

Although cervical stenosis appears as a major factor influencing pain during hysteroscopy to reduce the risk of false passage and perforation the best practice is to begin the hysteroscopic procedure without any sedation or general anesthesia in an operating room. The patient should be informed that any significant pain perceived

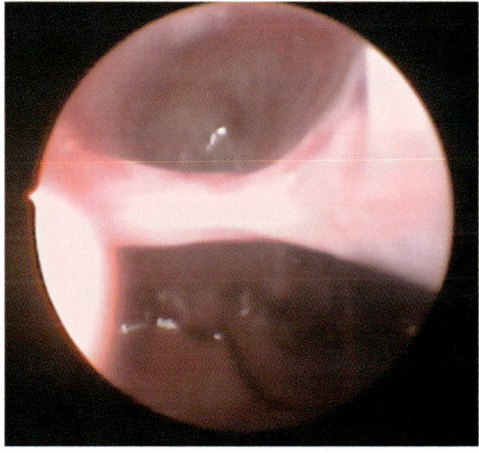

Fig. 7: False passage

and discomfort while the procedure is being carried out helps to avoid a false passage. Therefore, a sudden increase of patient's pain, the characteristic appearance of white/red tissue and non-visualization of any cervical gland opening are warning signs of a false passage into the cervical fibro-myometrial tissue. When a false passage or perforation are suspected the procedure should be abandoned. The patient should be given antibiotics and observed for 24 h in the hospital. If any other pelvic organ injury (e.g. bowel) is suspected, laparoscopy is needed, particularly when the injury occurs during active surgery involving the application of energy source.

Tips and tricks for a 28-year-old woman with primary infertility and cervical stenosis with previous false passage.

First step: *Before performing a new hysteroscopic procedure:*

Carefully perform a clinical evaluation defining the symptomatology: This 28-year-old woman was before and is at present with normal menses. Amenorrhea, cyclical lower abdominal discomfort and hematometra were and are not present after false passage caused by the previously hysteroscopic procedure.

Second step: *Before performing the new hysteroscopic procedure*:

Re-valuate the anatomy of pelvic organs: clinical bimanual examination and ultrasound evaluation may help to identify any anatomical modifications of the uterine axis and the angle between cervical canal and corpus.

Third step: *When to plan a new hysteroscopic procedure*:

Since menstrual bleedings are still present in this 28-year-old woman, we will plan during the menstrual flow. The menstrual bleeding helps to identified the correct direction. The orientation of the longitudinal crests "arbor vitae" and blood guide us into the cervical canal according to the principles of forward oblique scope. Since a clear way to the IO is sometime difficult to visualize, a mechanical scissors–graspers can be used to dilate with gentle manipulation of the cervical canal. Were repeatedly open and close the grasper jaws in the transverse plane with a slow progression of the scope to reach the IO and to pass into the uterine cavity.

Fourth step: *What to do after confirmation of the inability to access the uterine cavity in case of severe uterine malposition*

In case of an anteverted uterus combined with a severe degree of retroflexion, we straighten the uterine axis with a traction putting a tenaculum on the anterior lip of the cervix to make easier the progression of cope under ultrasound guide.

✍ Key Points

Action	Comments
1. Take an accurate medical, gynecologic, and obstetric history (pregnancies, dilation and curettage, cervical procedures that may increase the risk of cervical stenosis)	Identify risk factors for cervical stenosis in order to anticipate difficult navigation of the endocervical canal.
2. Perform a bimanual examination to assess uterine size and position and sound the uterus to determine its depth.	Assess cervical/uterine position to determine the direction in which the hysteroscope could be inserted because insertion of the hysteroscope can be the most difficult aspect of the procedure.
3. Entry into the cervical canal and uterine cavity under direct vision using gentle manipulation to minimize trauma according to the principles of forward oblique scope	Advance under hysteroscopic view minimizing trauma to the cervical canal
4. Apply a tenaculum to the anterior/posterior lip of the cervix	Help to straight the uterine axis and to immobilize the uterus
5. Avoid blind cervical dilatation (Hagar dilators or a lacrimal duct probe)	Use mechanical scissors–graspers to dilate with gentle manipulation the cervical canal under hysteroscopic view
6. Perform ultrasound evaluation and proceed under ultrasonographic guidance in selected procedures	Help to identify any anatomical modifications of the uterine axis and the angle between CC and corpus. Help to guide hysteroscope in difficult cases, e.g. when the patient has a history of false passage or uterine perforation
7. Opt for a smaller hysteroscope	Smaller scope will require less cervical dilation
8. Administer a paracervical block	Consider this option if hysteroscopic procedure is expected to be difficult, especially in women at risk of significant pain
9. Give misoprostol to prime the cervix	Consider giving 200–400 µg of intravaginal misoprostol 3 to 12 hours preoperatively to minimize cervical complications in selected cases.
10. Surgeon performing should have obtained basic competencies in order to perform effectively and safely complex hysteroscopies	Develop knowledge and aptitude to perform complex procedures under expert training.

BIBLIOGRAPHY

1. Ahmad G, Attarbashi S, O'Flynn H, Watson AJ. Pain relief in office gynecology: a systematic review and meta-analysis. Eur J ObstetGynecol Reprod Biol. 2011;155:3–13.

2. Al-Fozan H, Firwana B, Al Kadri H, Hassan S, Tulandi T. Preoperative ripening of the cervix before operative hysteroscopy. Cochrane Database of Systematic Reviews 2015, Issue 4.

3. American College of Obstetricians and Gynecologists. ACOG technology assessment in obstetrics and gynecology no. 13: hysteroscopy. Obstet Gynecol. 2018; 131: e151–e156.

4. Barbieri RL. Stenosis of the external cervical os: an association with endometriosis in women with chronic pelvic pain. FertilSteril 1998;70: 271–73.

5. Bettocchi S, Bramante S, Bifulco G, et al. Challenging the cervix: strategies to overcome the anatomic impediments to hysteroscopy: analysis of 31,052 office hysteroscopies. FertilSteril. 2016;105:e16–e17.

6. Bettocchi S, Selvaggi L. A vaginoscopic approach to reduce the pain of office hysteroscopy. J AmAssoc Gynecol Laparosc1997;4:255–8.

7. Choksuchat C. Clinical use of misoprostol in nonpregnant women: review article. J Minim Invasive Gynecol. 2010;17:449–55.

8. Cooper NA, Smith P, Khan KS, Clark TJ. Vaginoscopic approach to outpatient hysteroscopy: a systematic review of the effect on pain. BJOG.2010;117:532–39.

9. Guida M, Di Spiezio Sardo A, Acunzo G, Sparice S, Bramante, S, Piccoli, R, et al. Vaginoscopic versus traditional office hysteroscopy: a randomized controlled study. Hum Reprod. 2006;21: 3253–57.

10. Mazzon I, Favilli A, Horvath S, Grasso M, Di Renzo GC, Laurenti E, et al. Pain during diagnostic hysteroscopy: what is the role of the cervical canal? A pilot study. European Journal of Obstetrics and Gynecology and Reproductive Biology 2014;183:169–73.

11. Sagiv R, Sadan O, Boaz M, Dishi M, Schechter E, Golan A. A new approach to office hysteroscopy compared with traditional hysteroscopy: a randomized controlled trial. Obstet Gynecol 2006;108:387–92.

12. Shveiky D, Rojansky N, Revel A, Benshushan A, Laufer N, Shushan A Complications of hysteroscopic surgery: "Beyond the learning curve". J Minim Invasive Gynecol. 2007;14(2): 218.

13. Tasma ML, Louwerse MD, Hehenkamp WJ, Geomini PM, Bongers MY, Veersema S, et al. Misoprostol for cervical priming prior to hysteroscopy in postmenopausal and premenopausal nulliparous women; a multicenter randomised placebo controlled trial. BJOG. 2018;125:81–89.

Hemorrhage

Alappat Kurian Joseph

Hysteroscopic myomectomy was being performed for a 3 cm grade 2 fibroid and then there was massive Hemorrhage.

Uterine leiomyomas are tumors of the myometrium that have a prevalence as high as 70 to 80% at age 50. Myomas, are usually asymptomatic, but are associated with abnormal uterine bleeding (AUB) especially heavy menstrual bleeding (HMB), infertility and recurrent pregnancy loss.

FIGO uterine fibroid subclassification system defines, intracavitary lesions are attached to the endometrium by a narrow stalk and are classified as type 0, whereas types 1 and 2 require a portion of the lesion to be intramural—with type 1 having less than 50% involvement and type 2 at least 50% (Fig. 1).

Submucous myomas (types 0, 1, and 2) up to 4 to 5 cm diameter can be removed under hysteroscopic direction by experienced surgeons, whereas larger and multiple myomas are best removed abdominally. Type 2 myomas are more likely to require a multistaged procedure than types 0 and 1.

One of the greatest concerns to the hysteroscopic surgeon is the risk of perforation and bleeding.

Severe bleeding requiring intervention occurs at a rate of 0.5 to 1.9%. Mainly observed during forceful dilatation, deep ablation and vaporization.

Preoperative Preparations: What should have been done to Prevent this Disaster?

This is not a procedure to be attempted in an office setting for this size of the myoma. So the patient should be treated in an operation theater setting.

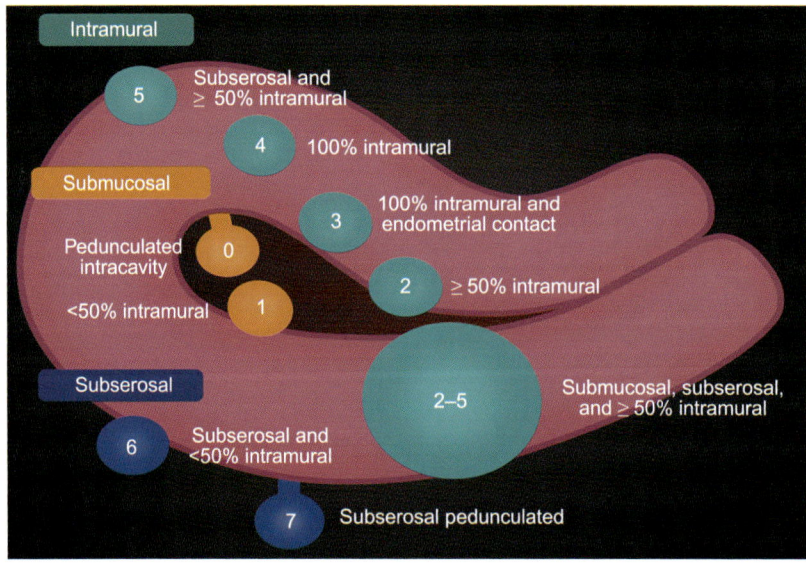

Fig. 1: FIGO uterine fibroid subclassification system

- Good history and proper diagnosis is the key to success. Previous surgeries may make the uterus adherent to the anterior abdominal wall, making a hysteroscopic procedure difficult.
- Check the size of the uterus and the myoma by good imaging ultrasound or MRI.
- Determine the correct size, number, location and the type A Grade 2 myoma may have a bigger extension into the myometrium. Proper classification is essential—STEP-W, FIGO—are all helpful. Major advantage of the STEPW classification is in its ability to group the submucous fibroids by score, identifying a group in which 100% of the myomectomies will be complete and another group in which some incomplete myomectomies will occur. This will permit the surgeon to plan and better prepare for the surgery, to better inform the patient prior to consenting to the procedure (Fig. 2).
- Decision making—the complete history and clinical picture of the patient has to be reviewed before making the decision to do a hysteroscopic myomectomy. Discuss the pros and cons with the patient. The result of the procedure may not result in complete control of the bleeding with other causes of AUB. Also consent for a

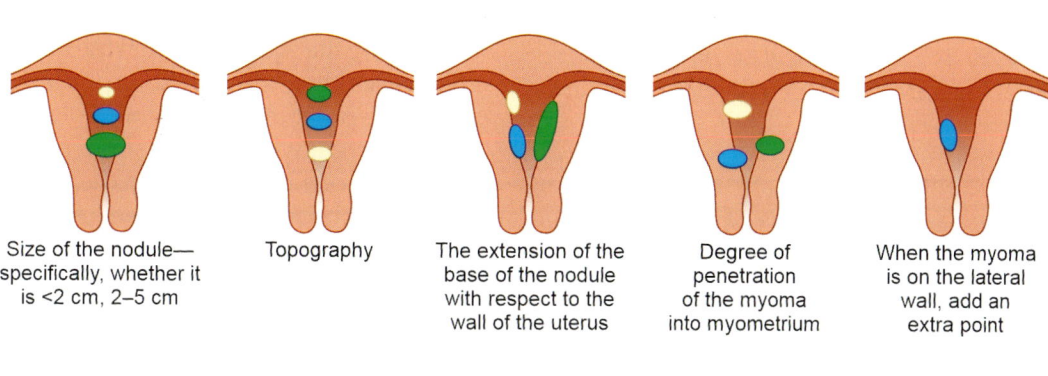

| Size of the nodule—specifically, whether it is <2 cm, 2–5 cm | Topography | The extension of the base of the nodule with respect to the wall of the uterus | Degree of penetration of the myoma into myometrium | When the myoma is on the lateral wall, add an extra point |

	Size (cm)	Topography	Extension of the base	Penetration	Lateral wall	Total
0	<2	Low	<1/3	0		
1	>2 – 5	Middle	>1/3–2/3	<50%	+1	
2	>5	Upper	>2/3	>50%		
Score	+	+	+	+	+	

How to score myoma using the STEP-W classification

	Total score	Group	Suggested treatment
○ = Score 0	0–4	I	Low-complexity hysteroscopic myomectomy
◔ = Score 1	5–6	II	Complex hysterocopic myomectomy. Consider giving a preoperative GnRH analog or performing a two-stage procedure, or both.
● = Score 2	6–9	III	Hysteroscopic approach is not recommended

Fig. 2: Lasmar's STEP-W scoring and predictability for successful myomectomy

2-stage procedure, associated laparoscopy or laparotomy should be taken anticipating problems.

- Steps to reduce the bleeding:
  - Preop GnRh to reduce the size and vascularity of the fibroid and gain time to improve the hematocrit of the patient.
  - Misoprostol—to soften the cervix and ease entry into the uterine cavity 100–200 g vaginally one hour before.
  - Vasopressin decreases bleeding during the procedure. Vasopressin 20 units in 50 ml saline, 10 to 15 ml is infiltrated around the cervix. Alert the anesthetic team when administering the injection.

Beware of the contraindications—Hysteroscopic surgery is contraindicated in active pelvic infection, intrauterine pregnancy, cervical or uterine malignancy.

Intraoperative Management of Hemorrhage (Figs 3 and Flowchart 1)

- Stabilise the patient
- Emergency supportive measures—call for help, check with anesthetic team—think of pulmonary embolism or edema, if vitals are stable, maintain the IV fluid line, organise for blood transfusion, use pressors if indicated, use tranexamic acid-1–2 g slow IV over 10 minutes.

- Restore the hysteroscopy image—check fluid input, note adequate pressure, see the output if working and if blood stained, if no picture seen and if perforation is not suspected, increase pressure up to 150 mm Hg.
- If image can not be restored and if bleeding persists—consider a perforation of the uterus, a sudden loss of vision with bleeding-prepare for laparoscopy/laparotomy.
- If image is restored attempt to identify the site of the bleeding—this is done with a judicious combination of increasing the intrauterine pressure, altering the inflow and outflow volumes. If the bleeding point is seen then try to decrease it by further increasing the pressure. When the bleeding decreases then attempt to coagulate the bleeding point using the monopolar—use a low current with a broad surface tip or a roller ball or a bipolar. When the bleeding stops watch for any other bleeding points.
- If myoma is seen partly resected attempt to complete the resection. The myoma may be intramural, then use methods like hydro-massage or bimanual massage to lever it out. If it goes deeper and cannot be removed consider a second procedure at a later date by which time most of it gets extruded.

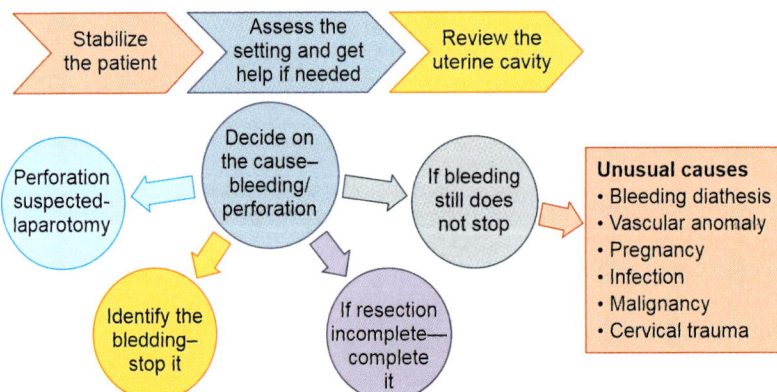

Fig. 3: Intraoperative management of Hemorrhage

Flowchart 1: Management—severe bleeding

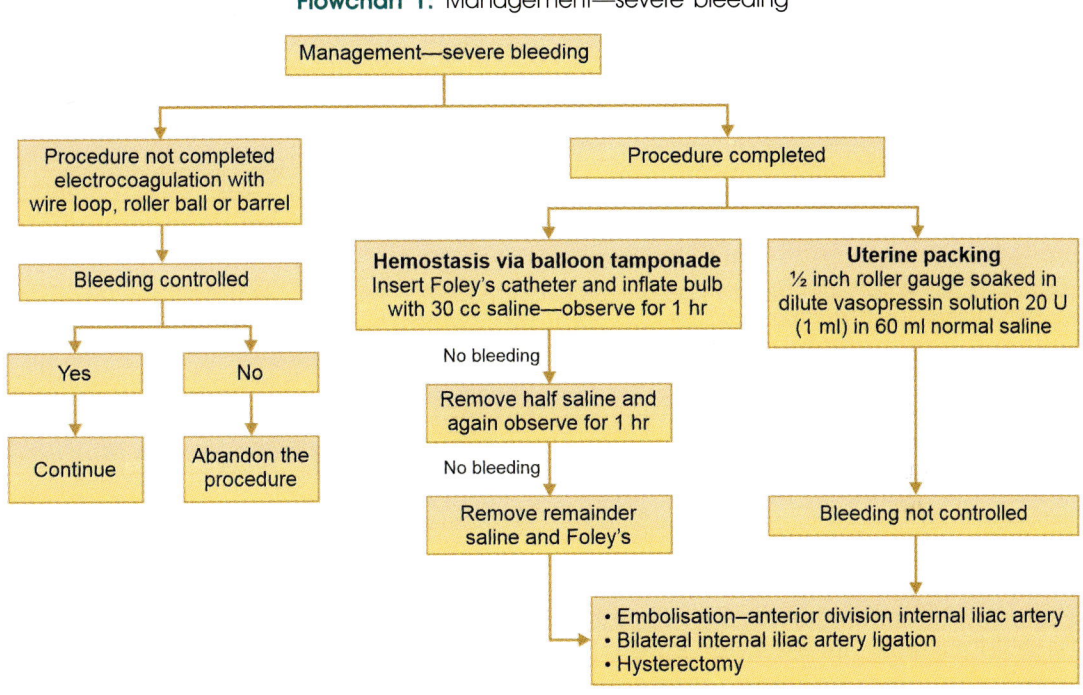

- If area is suspected to be adenomyotic—try to minimise the bleeding by coagulating with the bipolar. Wide coagulation around the site of bleeding will help to stop the bleeding. The thickness of the uterine wall may vary so better control is with bipolar.

- If the bleeding still does not stop think of the unusual causes of bleeding-AV malformation, an unsuspected pregnancy, malignancy. If entry was difficult withdraw the scope and check for lacerations on the cervical canal or a tear on the myometrium.

- If the bleeding is reduced intrauterine pressure could be applied using a No 14 or 16 Foleys catheter-depending on the size of the uterus, fluid is instilled till some resistance is felt-10–15 ml usually. The Foleys can cause postoperative pain and may need to be deflated to reduce the pain. The Foleys is kept for 24 hours and then removed. Once the bleeding is controlled check the haematocrit and the coagulation profile.

Postoperative management—support with hematinics. Do an ultrasound to verify completeness of the procedure.

Hysteroscopic myomectomy has definite indications and could be done in carefully selected cases only with a proper set up.

BIBLIOGRAPHY

1. AAGL Practice Report: Practice Guidelines for the Diagnosis and Management of Submucous Leiomyomas. Journal of Minimally Invasive Gynecology, Vol 19, No 2, March/April 2012.

2. Ingrid Pabinger, Tranexamic acid for treatment and prophylaxis of bleeding and hyperfibrinolysis. Wien Klin Wochenschr. 2017 May;129(9-10):303–316.

3. Linda D Bradley. Hysteroscopic Myomectomy, Uptodate 2019, Uptodate.com

4. Munro M, et al. Two FIGO system of classification of AUB. Int J of Gyn Obs; 2018: 1–16.

5. Ricardo Bassil Lasmar, Zhang Xinmei, Paul D. Indman, Roger Keller Celest, Attilio Di Spiezio Sardo. Feasibility of a new system of classification of submucous myomas: a multicenter study. Fertility and Sterility, Vol. 95, No. 6, May 2011.

Uterine Perforation

PG Paul

A 24-years-old P0A4 underwent hysteroscopic metroplasty for partial septate uterus and surgeon discovered uterine perforation.

Uterine septum is one of the commonest uterine anomalies and it is often associated with recurrent pregnancy loss (Fig. 1). Prevalence of the uterine septum ranges between 1 to 2 per 1,000 and as high as 15 per 1,000. Initially, uterine septa were believed to be predominantly fibrous tissue but biopsy specimens and magnetic resonance imaging (MRI) suggest that septa are composed primarily of muscle fibers and less connective tissue.

Hysteroscopic metroplasty is the accepted treatment modality in modern practice. Pregnancy wastage in women with septate uterus has been reported to decrease to half in women who undergo hysteroscopic septum incision. It can be performed with an operative hysteroscope using scissors or electrosurgery/ resectoscope. Hysteroscopic metroplasty can be performed as an outpatient procedure and generally accepted to be safe. However, complications like uterine perforation, hemorrhage, air embolism, fluid overload, pulmonary edema and infection can occur.

Preoperative Preparations

Risk of uterine perforation during septum incision can be reduced by appropriate preoperative evaluation. Careful differentiation between a septate uterus and bicornuate uterus. Rarely a combination of bicornuate uterus with subseptate uterus may be present.

- Hysterosalpingography is usually not confirmative, diagnostic accuracy of HSG ranges from 5.6 to 88%.
- 2D transvaginal ultrasonography can make a near accurate diagnosis of septate uterus (Fig. 2). But many sonologists report septate uterus as bicornuate uterus.

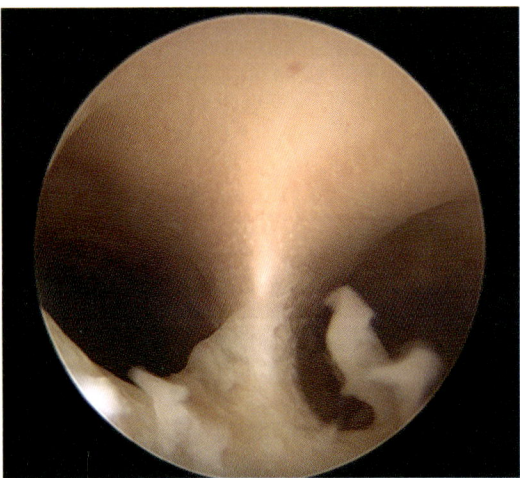

Fig. 1: Hysteroscopic view—septate uterus cat's eyes appearance

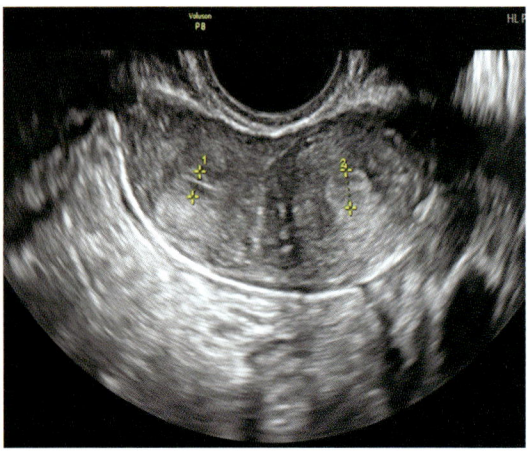

Fig. 2: Axial view of septate uterus on 2D TVS

- 3D transvaginal ultrasonography can confirm the diagnosis and also will show the extent and thickness of the septum (Fig. 3). MRI is indicated only when complex congenital anomaly is suspected.

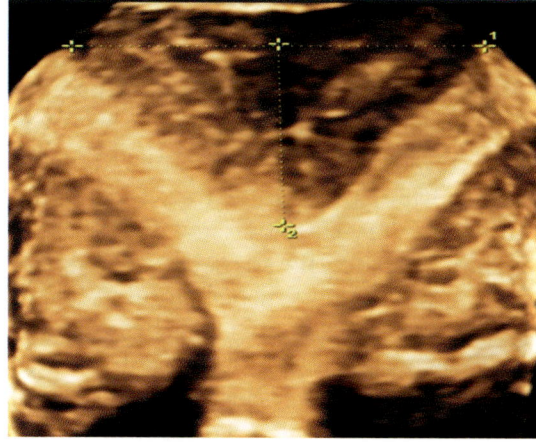

Fig. 3: Septate uterus on 3D TVS

American Society for Reproductive Medicine (ASRM) Criteria for the Diagnosis of Normal or Septate Uterus (Fig. 4)

- **Normal or arcuate uterus:** Depth from the interstitial line to the apex of the indentation 90°.
- **Septate uterus:** Depth from the interstitial line to the apex of the indentation >1.5 cm and angle of the indentation 1 cm. Internal endometrial cavity is similar to a partial septate uterus.

ASRM: 2016 Guidelines for the Diagnosis

- There is fair evidence that 3-D ultrasound, sonohysterography, and MRI are good diagnostic tests for distinguishing a septate and bicornuate uterus when compared with laparoscopy/ hysteroscopy (Grade B).
- It is recommended that imaging with hysteroscopy should be used to diagnose uterine septa rather than laparoscopy with hysteroscopy because this approach is less invasive (Grade B).

Intraoperative Precautions

There is always a debate whether a laparoscopy should be performed simultaneously with hysteroscopic septum incision. Laparoscopy helps to confirm the shape of fundus before performing the septum incision. In cases of infertility, it is useful to evaluate other causes.

- Routine use of misoprostol for cervical dilatation is not required in these cases. In majority of cases no dilatation is required for operative hysteroscope or small resectoscope.
- Misoprostol use can make the cervix patulous and fluid leak around the hysteroscope, causing poor distention. Division of lower part of septum is usually difficult due to poor distention of the lower segment of uterus. The fluid leakage

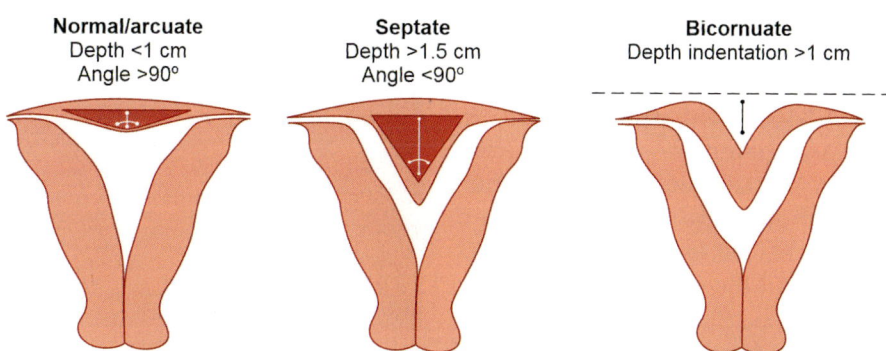

Fig. 4: ASRM criteria for diagnosis normal and septate uterus

can be reduced by applying a tenaculum or Gimpelson forceps over the cervix (Fig. 5).

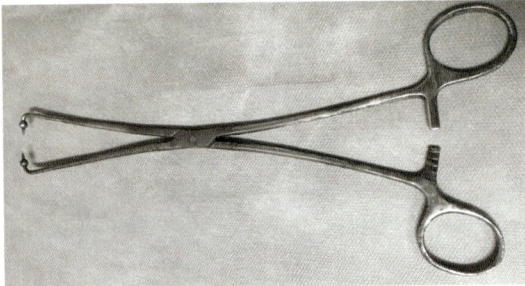

Fig. 5: Gimpelson forceps

- Instrument selection for hysteroscopic septum incision is important. Thin septa can be divided with a 5 mm Bettocchi hysteroscope and 7 Fr scissors. A pair of sharp scissors is required for fine cutting (Fig. 6).

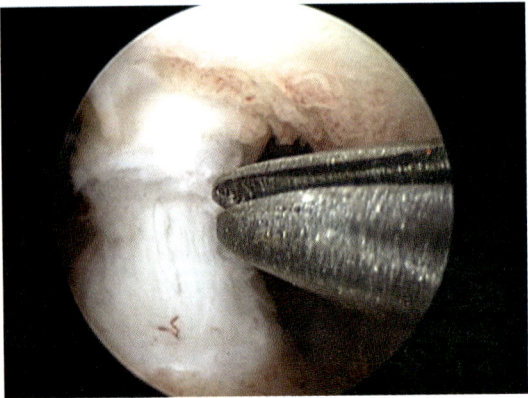

Fig. 6: Septoplasty with 5 Fr scissors

- Good visibility of uterine cavity and the septum during every step of hysteroscopic surgery is the key to successful septum incision. To ensure good visibility, appropriate distention of the uterine cavity has to be maintained. The distention medium should be kept clear and transparent before incising the septum and throughout the surgery.
- Maintaining good distention and visibility is sometimes difficult when the scissors is introduced into the operating channel.

Increasing the distention pressure can overcome this difficulty.

- Monopolar and bipolar electrodes can also be used instead of scissors, but moving the electrode sidewise and precise control of the incision is difficult especially for inexperienced hysteroscopist. We prefer small caliber (16.5/18 Fr) bipolar resectoscope with Collin's knife for thicker or complete septum.
- To remain midway of septum is another important precaution to avoid complication. Very close-up view of the septum can mislead the surgeon, so periodic panoramic view will be helpful. When the upper part of septum is reached, it will be wider and cutting systematically from left to right or vice versa is advisable (Fig. 7). Cutting more on one side and then doing the other side can be misleading.

Use of appropriate power setting for electrosurgical cutting is another safety precaution. Before starting the procedure, set the appropriate power adequate to cut the tissues without spark and at the same time apt enough to not allow electrode from sticking to the tissues. High power setting can cause uncontrolled cutting resulting in myometrial thinning or perforation.

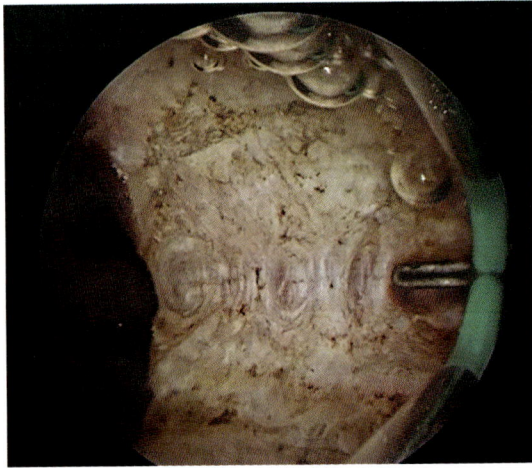

Fig. 7: Septoplasty of thicker septum with Collin's knife

- Most difficult decision making during surgery is deciding the end point of septum cutting. Simultaneous laparoscopic control for transillumination is misleading and unnecessary. Ideally, simultaneous transabdominal ultrasound examination is to be done to find the residual thickness of myometrium. In our practice we inspect the cavity from internal os and decide to cut the septum in the same level with both ostia (Fig. 8). There are reports of rupture uterus during pregnancy following septum incision even without perforation. Rule of thumb is undercutting, leaving residual septa of less than 1 cm.[3]

Di Spiezio introduced a noval instrument, 5 French graduated intrauterine palpator to measure the portion of the remaining septum (Fig. 9). In his Series of cases,

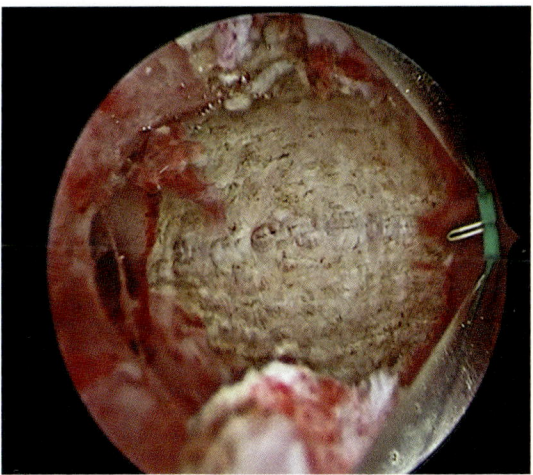

Fig. 8: Hysteroscopic view of uterine cavity after septal incision

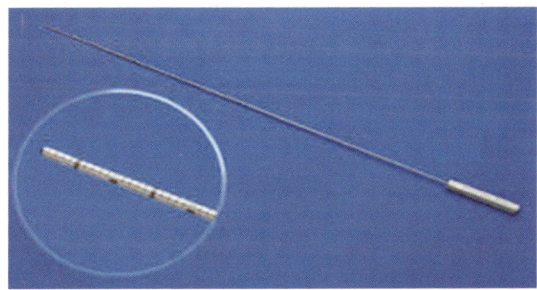

Fig. 9: Graduated intrauterine palpator

metroplasty was stopped when the intrauterine palpator showed that the resected septum corresponded to the presurgical ultrasonographic measures, and had a fundal notch of 1 cm. Mean procedural time was similar in the palpator and control groups (12.6 minutes *vs* 11.7 minutes) but more complete resections occurred in the palpator group than the control group (71 *vs* 41%), although the number of suboptimal resections was similar (28 *vs* 20%) (Flowchart 1).

Principles of Metroplasty

1. To horizontally divide the septum rather than excise the septum
2. Fundal myometrium should be at least 1.5 cm in depth
3. Postsurgery, IUCD insertion for at, least 3 months with estrogenisation is only recommended for wide or complete septa.

Diagnosis of Uterine Perforation

Following signs are useful to diagnose uterine perforation while performing hysteroscopic metroplasty.

1. Sudden loss of vision and collapse of uterine cavity while operating with previous good visibility. There may be associated bleeding at this time.
2. Loss of resistance with further movement of operating instrument.
3. Direct visualization of the uterine perforation site or abdominal organs like loops of intestine or pelvic side wall.
4. Consumption of large quantity of irrigation fluid. Peristaltic pump may work continuously to maintain intrauterine pressure

Any of these signs should alert the surgeon to suspect perforation. Final confirmation is by laparoscopy and direct visualization of perforation.

Management of Perforation (Fig. 9)

It depends on various factors like the type of instrument used for septum incision, size of

Flowchart 1: Management of perforation

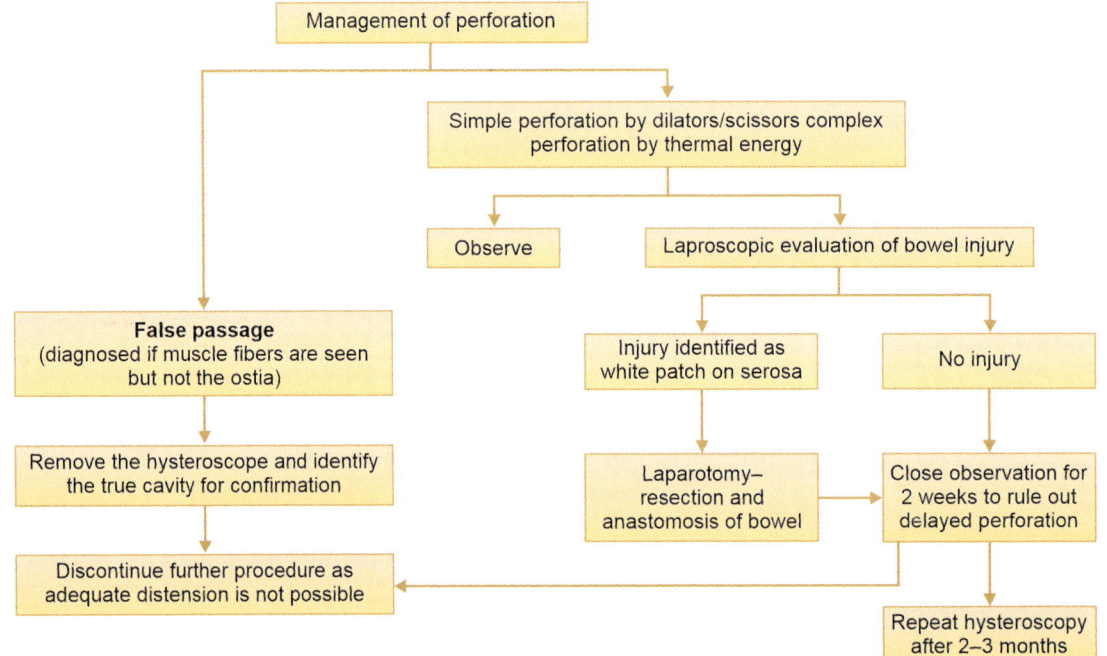

the perforation and the abdominal organs suspected to be injured. Unlike perforations for other operative hysteroscopic procedures, future pregnancy complication like rupture uterus has to be specifically addressed in our case scenario. Following points should be considered for choosing the management.

- If the perforation is small and occurred with hysteroscopic scissors towards the completion of septum incision, procedure is stopped and patient can be conservatively managed.
- If simultaneous laparoscopy has been performed, stop the hysteroscopy and assess the perforation laparoscopically.
- If the perforation has occurred with resectoscope and electrosurgery, apart from the uterine perforation, injury to vital organs has to be checked laparoscopically. If bowel adhesions to the uterus are suspected due to previous surgery, chances of bowel injury is likely. Laparoscopic inspection of rectosigmoid and systematic

evaluation of small bowel loops should be performed for any bowel burn, hematoma or bleeding. Bladder and iliac vessels can be injured, although rare, therefore to be inspected.

There are many reports of uterine rupture in subsequent pregnancies following uterine perforation during septum incision. Considering this risk, it is better to repair all perforations laparoscopically. Technique of repairing uterine perforation is similar to laparoscopic myomectomy closure. Usually single layer closure is sufficient as perforations are small. Coagulating the site of perforation should not be performed as it can result in poor healing.

If the septum incision is not completed while the perforation occurred, it can be completed after laparoscopic suturing. Any injury or diathermy blanching of vital organs should be assessed and repaired if necessary.

Sometimes large quantity of irrigation fluid can be present in the peritoneal cavity which can be sucked out during laparoscopy.

Other suggested practical tip is to feel the fundus with Collins knife for the resistance. We do not find this useful. If you encounter active bleeders during cutting, it suggests that myometrium is being cut and probably have to stop at that point.

Another usual problem that happens towards the end of septum incision is contraction of uterus causing distortion of the cavity. This happens when you reduce the pressure towards the end of surgery allowing the uterus to contract. So never change the pressure in between the surgery, rather keep it steady throughout cutting.

American Society for Reproductive Medicine (ASRM) 2016

Recommendations: Summary

- There is insufficient evidence to conclude that a uterine septum is associated with infertility (Grade C).
- Hysteroscopic septum incision is associated with improved clinical pregnancy rates in women with infertility (Grade C).
- Fair evidence that a uterine septum contributes to miscarriage and preterm birth (Grade B).
- Some evidence suggests that a uterine septum may increase the risk of other adverse pregnancy outcomes such as malpresentation, intrauterine growth restriction, placental abruption, and perinatal mortality (Grade B).
- Some limited studies indicate that hysteroscopic septum incision is associated with a reduction in subsequent miscarriage rates and improvement in live-birth rates in patients with a history of recurrent pregnancy loss (Grade C).
- Some limited studies indicate that hysteroscopic septum incision is associated with an improvement in live-birth rate in women with infertility or prior pregnancy loss (Grade C).

- There is insufficient evidence to conclude that obstetric outcomes are different when comparing the size as defined by length or width of uterine septa (Grade C).
- There is insufficient evidence to recommend a specific method for hysteroscopic septum incision (Grade C).
- Although the available evidence suggests that the uterine cavity is healed by 2 months postoperatively, there is insufficient evidence to advocate a specific length of time before a woman should conceive (Grade C).
- There is insufficient evidence for or against recommending danazol or GnRH agonists to thin the endometrium prior to hysteroscopic septum incision (Grade C).
- There is insufficient evidence to recommend for or against adhesion prevention treatment, or any specific method following hysteroscopic septum incision (Grade C).

✍ Key Points

1. Hysteroscopic septum incision is an accepted treatment for septate uterus.
2. It can be performed as an outpatient procedure with low complication rate.
3. Perforation of uterus is rare complication which needs proper management.
4. Perforation is suspected when there is sudden loss of visibility—other signs are visualization of pelvic organs like bowel loops.
5. Confirmation and management requires laparoscopy.
6. Laparoscopic suturing of the myometrial defect is similar to myomectomy.
7. Prevention of uterine perforation depends on precise diagnosis of septum and use of standard surgical techniques.

BIBLIOGRAPHY

1. Di Spiezio Sardo A, Zizolfi B, Bettocchi S, Exacoustos C, Nocera C, Nazzaro G, da Cunha Vieira M, Nappi C. Accuracy of Hysteroscopic

Metroplasty With the Combination of Presurgical 3-Dimensional Ultrasonography and a Novel Graduated Intrauterine Palpator: A Randomized Controlled Trial. J Minim Invasive Gynecol. 2016 May-Jun;23(4):557–66.

2. Fedele L, Bianchi S, Marchini M, Mezzopane R, Di Nola G, Tozzi L. Residual uterine septum of less than 1 cm after hysteroscopic metroplasty does not impair reproductive outcome. Hum Reprod. 1996; 11(4): 727–9.

3. Grimbizis GF, Gordts S, Sardo AD, Brucker S, DeAngelis C, Gergolet M, et al. The ESHRE/ESGE consensus on the classification of female genital tract congenital anomalies. Hum Reprod 2013;28:2032–44.

4. Judith FW Rikken, Claudia R KowalikMark H Emanuel, Ben Willem J Mol,Fulco Van der Veen, Madelon van Wely. Septum resection for women of reproductive age with a septate uterus. Cochrane Database of Systematic Reviews 2017.

5. Rafael F. Valle RF, Ekpo GE. Hysteroscopic Metroplasty for the Septate Uterus: Review and Meta-Analysis. JMIG. 2013; 20(1): 22–42.

6. Satiroglu H, et al. Uterine rupture at the 29th week of subsequent pregnancy after hysteroscopic resection of uterine septum. Fertil steril. 2009; 91(3): 934.e1–3.

7. Uterine septum: a guideline Practice Committee of the American Society for Reproductive Medicine American Society for Reproductive Medicine, Birmingham, Alabama. Fertility and Sterility. 2016 Volume 106, Issue 3; pp 530–540.

8. Uterine septum: a guideline. Practice Committee of the American Society FOR Reproductive Medicine. FertilSteril. 2016 Sep 1;106(3):530–40.

9. Valle RF, Ekpo GE. Hysteroscopic metroplasty for the septate uterus: review and meta-analysis. J Min Invas Gynecol 2013;20:22–42.

Case 4

Saline Media induced Operative Hysteroscopy Intravascular Absorption (OHIA) Syndrome or Glycine Media induced Gynecological TURP Syndrome

Péter Török, Richa Sharma, Rahul Manchanda

A 32-years-old P1L1, known case of chronic renal disease, Underwent hysteroscopic adhesiolysis for severe Asherman's syndrome. Her BP was normal during postoperative period but had developed repeated episodes of vomiting, headache and blurring of vision.

DIAGNOSIS

Saline media induced—operative hysteroscopy intravascular absorption (OHIA) syndrome or glycine media induced gynecological TURP syndrome.

INTRODUCTION

There is a spectrum of adverse events associated with operative hysteroscopy and the frequency of complications are reported to be as low as 0.24% but may go up to 10% with more complicated surgeries like hysteroscopic metroplasty or myomectomy. Absorption of small amounts (1–2 L) occurs in 5–10% of patients with a mild, easily overlooked TUR syndrome, while the classic syndrome develops in <1% with intravascular absorption in excess of 2 liters. Severe TUR syndrome following 1.5% glycine absorption is associated with a mortality of 25%. The clinical presentation of glycine toxicity and hyponatremia may be difficult to distinguish from sepsis or DIC, and usually manifests 30–45 min after completion of surgery.

Currently with the use of saline as distension media, the incidence of fluid overload and dyselectrolytemia during operative hysteroscopy is less than 5%. Monopolar electrosurgical device require non-electrolyte solution (e.g. glycine) for distending the uterine cavity, while bipolar electrosurgical device can work with saline.

BSGE/ESGE 2018 defines fluid overload as:

- **Hypotonic** solution: Overload-fluid deficit threshold of **1000 ml** in healthy women of reproductive age and **750 ml** for elderly women or with cardiac and renal co-morbidities.
- **Isotonic** solution: Overload-fluid deficit threshold of **2500 ml** in healthy women of reproductive age and **1500 ml** for elderly women or with cardiac and renal co-morbidities.

Maintenance of fluid balance is a crucial part of every hysteroscopic surgery. Inflow and outflow of the fluid should be measured and fluid deficit should be calculated continuously. Appropriate intrauterine pressure should be maintained avoiding too high pressure, but having good visual conditions.

Several types of fluid delivery system are available in the market (Fig. 1). This includes Mounir's Pumpino, which is a simple and low cost novel office hysteromat, to the advanced innovations, like Hysteromat EASI® (Figs 2 and 3), an endoscopic automatic system for irrigation that is an intelligent, pressure-controlled double roller pump.

Preoperative Consideration

Factors Influencing the Absorption of Distension Fluid

1. **Hypotonic electrolyte-free solutions:** Intravazation of the distending fluid can cause several complications, depending on the type and amount of the fluid. Glycine, mannitol and sorbitol cause serious fluid overload.

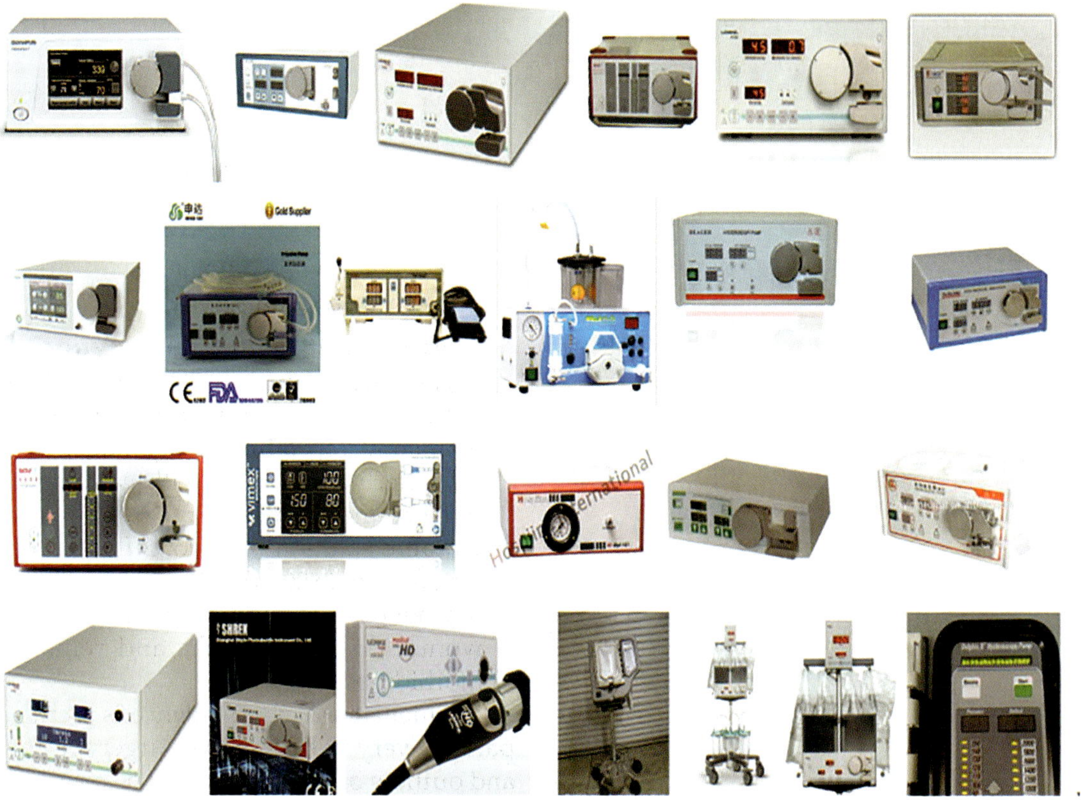

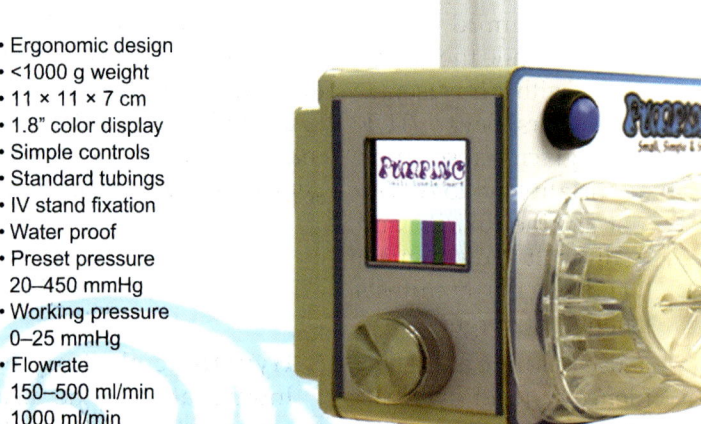

Fig. 1: Varieties for irrigating uterine cavity

- Ergonomic design
- <1000 g weight
- 11 × 11 × 7 cm
- 1.8" color display
- Simple controls
- Standard tubings
- IV stand fixation
- Water proof
- Preset pressure
  20–450 mmHg
- Working pressure
  0–25 mmHg
- Flowrate
  150–500 ml/min
  1000 ml/min
- Counter to 9999 ml

Fig. 2: Mounir's Pumpino

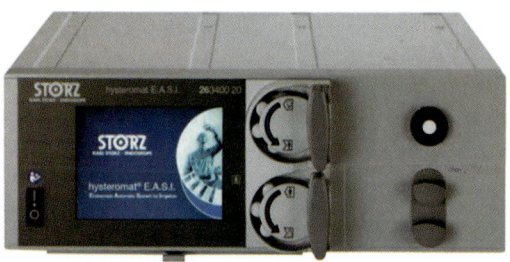

Fig. 3: Hysteromat EASI®

2. **Intrauterine pressures:** The higher the intrauterine pressure used, the higher the chance for intravazation of the fluid. Difference between intrauterine pressure and mean arterial pressure is important. The bigger the difference the higher chance of intravazation.

   • Intrauterine pressures of more than 75 mm Hg increases the volume of media entering the peritoneal cavity via fallopian tubes.

   • Intrauterine pressures > mean arterial pressure (normal 70 to 110 mmHg) especially in elderly and cardiac-renal co-morbidities also increases intravazation of the distending fluid.

3. **Size of uterine cavity and depth of myometrial penetration:** Surgeries affecting myometrium can damage vessels increasing the chance of fluid intravazation. The deeper surgery affects the myometrium and the thicker vessels could be damaged. Similarly the bigger surface of surgery (bigger uterus and uterine cavity), causes more vessels injuries. Large blood vessels breached and large myometrial surface area exposed (e.g. myomectomies) facilitates the absorption of fluid under pressure.

4. **Duration of surgery:** The longer the procedure, the more time for fluid to accumulate within the body. Duration should be decreased and optimized with proper skills, instrumentation and appropriate interventions, especially during myomectomies (GI and GII fibroids) endomyometrial resections, deep and wide

septum resections, difficult Asherman's metroplasties.

5. **Accelerated systemic fluid absorption occurs in:** Premenopausal patients have a higher risk of developing neurological complications. Cardiovascular, renal disease and elderly women are less likely to adapt to sudden significant increases in intravascular fluid.

Intraoperative Monitoring of Fluid Deficit

Measuring and recording the inflow of the distending medium is the easiest part of the procedure. By following the container of the fluid it can be clearly seen the exact volume of the fluid has been used. If an automated circulating system is used, it will show on the display continuously the consumed fluid volume. Modern systems can be set to alarm on a predefined value.

Measuring and recording the outflow is not as simple as the inflow. Outflowing fluid can be gathered in a bag and can be measured. During manipulation, withdrawal and insertion the scope, distension medium can be spread around, so the amount in the bag will be not precise. Using circulating system the exact volume of the outflowing solution will be recorded.

Fluid deficit calculated by subtracting the outflow volume from the inflow. Amount of fluid on the drapes (can be measured by scale) and in the abdominal cavity (disseminated through the Fallopian tubes, can be detected by transvaginal ultrasonography) should be always kept in mind.

Tips for Monitoing Fluid Deficit

• Closed systems should be used as they allow more accurate measurement of the fluid output (Fig. 4).

• Drapes that contain a fluid reservoir or the devices that sucks fluid from the ground should be used (Fig. 5).

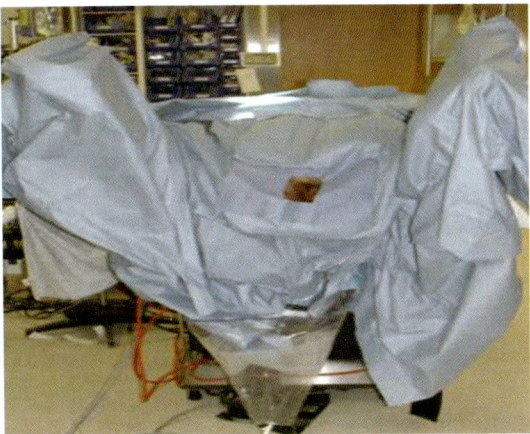

Fig. 4: Drapes with pouch—collects fluid

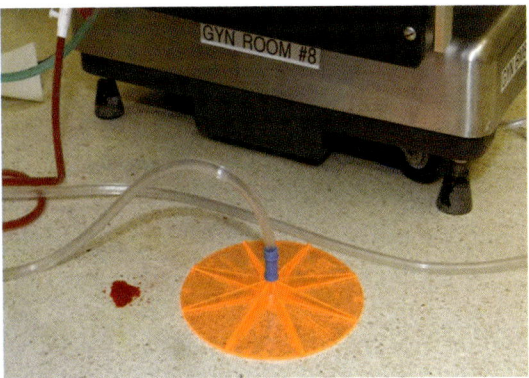

Fig. 5: Puddle Vac AKA "Sucky Ducky"

- Automated fluid measurement systems are more accurate.
- Theater team should keep fluid deficit balance **every 10 min** and at the end of each fluid bag used.

In case of any sign of fluid overload detected during surgery, it must be stopped immediately. Inflow and outflow of the fluid should always be monitored and regulated (Fig. 6). Strict adherence to BSGE/ESGE inflow and outflow chart can alleviate the possibility of fluid overload (Fig. 7).

Postoperative Management

Signs of hyponatremia and hypotonic status should be carefully observed. Symptoms usually develop when concentration of serum sodium drops below 125 mmol/L.

Sign of fluid overload detected
↓
Interrupt surgery
- Check for signs, mental status
- Evaluate hemodynamic status
- Laboratory tests: Hematocrit, platelets, blood urea nitrogen, creatinine, sodium, potassium, bicarbonate, chloride, glucose, ammonia (glycine is metabolized to ammonia), and plasma osmolality

Fig. 6: Introperative management

The most frequent symptoms are headache, nausea, vomiting and weakness. With more fluid intravazation, the osmotic imbalance will shift water in intracellular and interstitial spaces causing brain edema and increased intracranial pressure. Signs like agitation, apprehension, confusion, weakness, nausea, vomiting, visual disturbances, blindness and headache can be observed. In more severe cases it can lead to brain stem herniation, coma and death. Serum level of sodium below 120 mmol/L may lead to confusion, lethargy, seizures, coma, arrhythmias, bradycardia and respiratory arrest (Table 1).

Management of Fluid Overload and Electrolyte Imbalance

1. General treatment includes monitoring and correction of fluid balance using urinary catheter. Intensive care unit (ICU) should be available.
2. Asymptomatic hyponatremia needs no special therapy. Fluid restriction and loop diuretics (e.g. furosemide) should be used. If overload is not verified, loop diuretics are contraindicated.
3. Hypertonic saline is indicated for symptomatic patients with hyponatremia and reduced serum osmolality or cerebral edema.
4. Patients with severe neurologic symptoms, marked hyponatremia, and minimally reduced serum osmolality or patients with renal disease: Hemodialysis can correct

BSGE/ESGE Recommended inflow and outflow chart

Date _____

Operation _____

Surgeon _____

Anesthetist _____

Energy of resectoscpe _____

Fluid medium used _____

Method of limiting intrauterine pressure:

Gravity   height above patient _____ meters

Pressure bag   maximum pressure used _____ mmHg

Automated system   brand _____

Method of monitoring distension fluid in theatre

Sole person identified to monitor fluid deticit, measuerd every 10 min	yes	☐	no	☐
Drape used with fluid reservoir	yes	☐	no	☐
Closed system, i.e. fluid collection with suction	yes	☐	no	☐

Operation start time	Fluid Input	Fluid Output	Fluid Balance
+10 min			
+20 min			
+30 min			
Review: If not likely to complete procedure in under 60 min consider stopping			
+40 min			
+50 min			
Review: Consider stopping procedure at 60 min			
Length of procedure min	Final	Final	Final

STOP procedure if fluid deficit reaches 1000 ml Hypotonic Solution (750 ml if elderly or with co-morbidities) or 2500 ml Isotonic Solution (1500 ml if elderly or with co-morbidities)

Fig. 7: Introperative monitoring of inflow and outflow chart

hyponatremia, volume expansion, and also remove the nonelectrolyte solute.

5. *Multidisciplinary approach*
   - Involvement of anesthetists, physicians and intensivists in an intensive care unit.
   - Strict fluid balance during intraoperative and postoperative period.

- Urinary catheterization and input-output charting.
- Frequent (hourly) oxygen saturations, electrolytes, calcium, urea and creatinine monitoring.
- Echocardiogram and chest X-ray (if signs of cardiac failure or pulmonary edema).

Table 1: Fluid overload and management			
Fluid overload	**Sodium concentration**	**Symptoms**	**Management**
Asymptomatic hyponatremia	125–135 mEq/L Osmolality normal 280 mOsm/L	—	Fluid restriction <1 lit/day and loop diuretics, e.g. furosamide
Symptomatic hyponatremia	125–120 mEq/L	Headache, nausea, vomiting and weakness Signs of cerebral irritation-agitation, apprehension, confusion, weakness, visual disturbances, blindness If significant-leads to coma and death	Multidisciplinary approach*
	<120 mEq/L	Confusion, lethargy, seizures, coma, arrhythmias, bradycardia and respiratory arrest	

*Recommended target increase of the serum Na^+ is 6 mmol/L over 24 h until 130 mmol/L is reached

- 100 ml bolus of 3% saline over 10 min and repeat up to 3 times followed by, slow IV infusion of 3% hypertonic sodium chloride infusion (typically 1–2 mmol/l/h to prevent pontine myelinolysis) until serum Na^+/> 125 mmol/L
- Sorbitol 3% (hypotonic sugar) can lead to hyperglycemia, hypocalcemia and myoclonus within an hour. Monitoring of the blood sugars and giving insulin according to sliding scale. Hypocalcemia must be corrected with 3 g of calcium gluconate over 10 min.

BSGE/ESGE 2018 Executive Committee —Safety Recommendations

- Isotonic, electrolyte—containing distension media such as normal saline should be used with mechanical instrumentation and bipolar electrosurgery because of low risk of hyponatremia and fluid overload
- Hypotonic, electrolyte-free distension media such as glycine and sorbitol should only be used with monopolar electrosurgical instruments.
- Carbon dioxide gaseous media should be used for diagnostic hysteroscopy only.

- Automated pressure delivery systems provides constant intrauterine pressure and accurate fluid deficit surveillance, advantageous in prolonged operative procedures.
- Measurement of the fluid deficit should be done at a minimum of 10 min intervals
- Local anesthesia with sedation should be considered for performing operative hysteroscopic procedures rather than general anesthesia.

✍ Key Points

1. Saline media induced—operative hysteroscopy Intravascular Absorption (OHIA) syndrome or glycine media induced gynecological TURP syndrome are most life threatening complications of distension media.
2. With the use of saline as distension media, the incidence of fluid overload and dyselectrolytemia during operative hysteroscopy is less than 5%.
3. Proper preoperative diagnosis, indication and evaluating the risk factors are important tools in term of succeeding the procedure.
4. Surgeon's skills and proper technique are most vital.

5. Continuous monitoring of distension media in and outflow is mandatory

6. Immediate recognition of fluid deficit and early diagnoses of fluid overload and hyponatremia with the prompt start of treatment (fluid balance, electrolyte balance, multidisciplinary team and in serious cases ICU available if needed) can avoid the severity of complications.

BIBLIOGRAPHY

1. AasEng MK, Langebrekke A, Hudelist G. Complications in operative hysteroscopy is prevention possible? Acta Obstet Gynecol Scand 2017? 96:1399.

2. Ciebiera M, £oziñski T, Wojtya C, Rawski W, Jakiel G. Complications in modern hysteroscopic myomectomy. Ginekol Pol. 2018;89(7): 398–404.

3. Hahn RG. Fluid absorption in endoscopic surgery. Br J Anaesth. 2006;96:8–20.

4. Istre O. Managing bleeding, fluid absorption and uterine perforation at hysteroscopy. Best Pract Res Clin Obstet Gynaecol. 2009; 23(5): 619–629.

5. Munro MG, Christianson LA. Complications of Hysteroscopic and Uterine Resectoscopic Surgery. Clin Obstet Gynecol. 2015; 58(4): 765–797.

6. Navdeep Sethi, Ravindra Chaturvedi, and Krishna Kumar. Operative hysteroscopy intra-vascular absorption syndrome: A bolt from the blue. Indian J Anaesth 2012 Mar-Apr; 56(2): 179–182.

7. Sethi N, Chaturvedi R, Kumar K. Operative hysteroscopy intravascular absorption syndrome: A bolt from the blue. Indian J Anaesth. 2012;56:179–82.

8. Umranikar S, Clark TJ, Saridogan E, et al. British Society for Gynaecological Endoscopy / European Society for Gynaecological Endoscopy Guideline Development Group for Management of Fluid Distension Media in Operative Hys-teroscopy. BSGE/ESGE guideline on manage-ment of fluid distension media in operative hysteroscopy. Gynecol Surg. 2016; 13(4): 289–303.

9. Verbalis JG, Goldsmith SR, Greenberg A, Korzelius C, Schrier RW, Sterns RH, Thompson CJ. Diagnosis, evaluation, and treatment of hyponatremia: expert panel recommenda-tions. Am J Med 2013; 126(10):S1–S42.

Air Embolism

Ashish Ramchandra Kale, Richa Sharma, Rahul Manchanda

40-year-old lady undergoing myoma resection and developed shortness of breath and sudden fall in saturation to 60% **Diagnosis—air embolism**

Uterine fibroids and uterine anatomy are an unique issue in gynecology for ages. With emerging theories and treatment modalities fibroids have always posed a different and difficult times for clinicians and surgeons. The management has changed over time with patient's desire and quality of life being the top most priority. Disscussion with the patient, about all the available options and then coming to a conclusion is the crux of today's practice. 2D or 3D TVS is the gold standard for mapping and localising the myomas.

Indications for Transcervical Resection of Myoma (TCRM)

- Types 0, 1, 2 submucus myomas up to 5 cm
- Patients wanting to avoid hysterectomy
- To preserve future fertility
- Prior to ART

Clinically significant air embolism is rare but potentially a fatal complication of operative hysteroscopy.

The incidence of fatal embolism is around 3 per 17,000 procedures, with mortality as high as 46%. However, the cut off point between the occurrence of major catastrophic episode and subtle but unequivocally important symptoms is yet undefined.

Signs of gas embolism: Sudden fall in oxygen saturation, hypotension, hypercarbia, arrhythmias, tachypnea, or a "mill wheel" murmur (characteristic splashing auscultatory sound). Immediate termination of the surgical procedure and a vigilant anesthesiologist's timely intervention is crucial in reducing the morbidity and mortality (Flowchart 1).

Etiologies for Air Embolism during Operative Hysteroscopy

- Increased volume of fluid used for distention.
- Extensive cervical dilatation, the risk of air embolism is higher.
- Removal and re-introduction of the hysteroscope may facilitate air entry into the vascular compartment, by causing "piston-like" transmission of air into the uterus.
- Air bubbles in the tubing of irrigation solution entering open venous sinuses under pressure or venous absorption of the bubbles produced by the vaporization of tissue.
- Residual debris and blood clots can also enter open venous sinuses under high-pressure irrigating solution.
- Inappropriate insufflation equipment can drive gas into the intravascular space such as when a laparoscopic CO_2 insufflator (maximum insufflation rate: 16 L/min) is inadvertently used instead of a hysteroscopic CO_2 insufflator (maximum insufflation rate: 100 ml/min).
- If the patient is in Trendelenburg position, the pressure differential between the endometrial cavity and the right heart can cause passage of air from the endometrial cavity to the uterine veins and subsequently the systemic venous circulation.

Preoperative Precautions

- Proper patient selection, fibroid mapping, proper instrumentation and good surgical expertise.
- Place the patient in dorsal lithotomy and avoid steep Trendelenburg position because it keeps the uterus above the level of heart and creates a venous vacuum with each diastolic relaxation.
- Preoperative cervical priming must be considered and minimize the cervical trauma.
- Use of GnRH agonists Preoperatively, narrow venous sinuses and help prevent this complication.

Intraoperative Precautions

- Use Vaginoscopic method and avoid using heavy weighted speculums and dilators.
- Intracervical injection of dilute vasopressin prior to dilatation of the cervix creates vascular spasm and may help prevent gas from entering the circulation.
- The American Association of Gynecologic Laparoscopists advocates the use of automated fluid pump and monitoring system. Measurement of the fluid deficit should be done at a minimum of 10 min intervals during hysteroscopic surgery.

- Flush System with fluid to remove air bubbles.
- Avoid using gas producing electrosurgical equipment as far as possible.
- Always keep the os occluded so as to prevent entry of room air. Keep the last dilator inside till resectoscope is assembled. Whenever electrode is to be changed keep the obturator inside.
- Avoid repetitive removal and reinsertion of the resectoscope (often seen during myoma resection). Best alternative is to use **Myosure device or TruClear device** that combines both resection and suction simultaneously.
- Maximum uterine distension pressure of 200 mmHg and maximum CO_2 flow rate of 100 ml/min.
- Anesthetist should closely monitor end tidal CO_2 (expired CO_2 measurement of each breath amounts to non-invasive estimation of $PaCO_2$) and can diagnose air embolism early.
- Where feasible, the use of local anesthesia with sedation should be considered for performing operative hysteroscopic procedures rather than general anesthesia because fluid overload may be minimised.

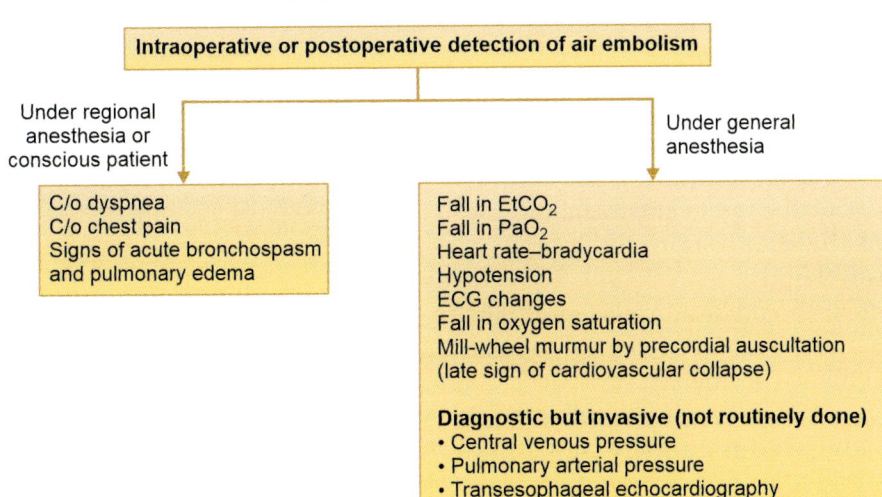

Flowchart 1: Detection of air embolism

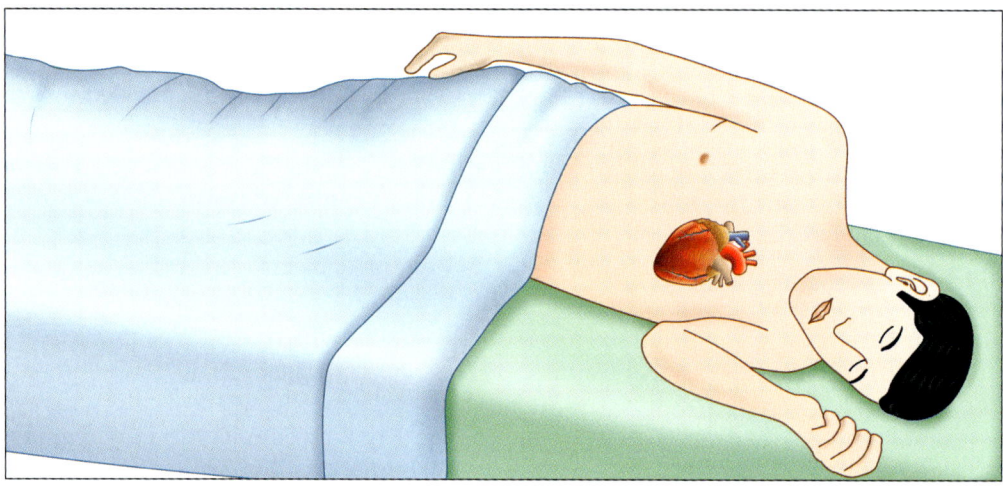

Fig. 1: Durant maneuver

The resultant pulmonary hypertension caused hypoxia, pulmonary vasoconstriction, and increased vascular permeability resulting in a drop in PET CO_2. This is the most important sign of intraoperative embolism, especially when accompanied by a decrease in blood pressure.

Management

- Immediately abandon the procedure.
- Irrigation fluid pressure should be released.
- The location of suspected gas entry should be identified and closed, which generally means removing any instrument from the uterus and clamping closed the cervical canal.
- The patient should be placed in "Durant maneuver"—left lateral position with head low and Trendelenburg position. As this elevates, the right ventricle above the level of the diaphragm and prevents embolism (Fig. 1).
- The patient should be administered 100% oxygen and insertion of central venous line should be considered.
- If hypovolemia is suspected, infuse intravenous fluids to increase central venous pressure.

- Inotropes and vasopressors should be used as required to maintain vital organ perfusion.
- Keep the central venous catheterization set ready to retrieve the air from the right ventricle outflow in case of cardiac arrest or persistent hemodynamic instability.
- Inotropic support and cardiopulmonary resuscitation should be instituted as necessary. Hyperbaric oxygen has been advised but its role in the treatment is debatable and it is not widely available.

✍ Key Points

1. The incidence of fatal air embolism is around 3 per 17,000 procedures, with mortality as high as 46%.
2. Preoperative cervical priming must be considered and minimize the cervical trauma.
3. Use of GnRH agonists preoperatively, narrow venous sinuses and help prevent this complication.
4. The American Association of Gynecologic Laparoscopists advocates the use of automated fluid pump and monitoring system. Measurement of the fluid deficit should be done at a minimum of 10 min intervals during hysteroscopic surgery
5. Avoid repetitive removal and reinsertion of the resectoscope or use Myosure or Trueclear

device that combines both resection and suction simultaneously.

6. Anesthetist should closely monitor end tidal CO_2 (expired CO_2 measurement of each breath amounts to non invasive estimation of $PaCO_2$) and can diagnose air embolism early.

7. Immediately abandoning the procedure, placing the patient in Durant maneuver and administering 100% oxygen are life saving measures.

BIBLIOGRAPHY

1. Baggish M, Brill A, Rosenweig B,Barbot J, Indman P. Fatal acute glycine and sorbitol toxicity during operative hysteroscopy. J Gynecol Surg 1993; 9(3):137–143.

2. Istre O, Bjoennes J, Naess R, Hornbaek K, Forman A. Postoperative cerebral edema after transcervical endometrial resection and uterine irrigation with 1.5% glycine. Lancet 1994; 344: 1187–1189.

3. Kaijser J, Roelofs HJM, Breimer LTM, Kooi SG. Excessive fluid overload with severe hyponatremia, cardiac failure, an cerebral edema complicating hysteroscopic myomectomy. JPelvic Med Surg 2007; 13:367–373.

4. Lee JW (2010) Fluid and electrolyte disturbances in critically ill patients. Electrolyte Blood Press 2010;8(2):72–81.

5. Sameer Umranikar and T. Justin Clark and Ertan Saridogan and Dimitrios Miligkos1 and Kirana Arambage and Emma Torbe and Rudi Campo and Attilio Di Spiezio Sardo and Vasilios Tanos and Grigoris Grimbizis and British Society for Gynaecological Endoscopy/European Society for Gynaecological Endoscopy Guideline Development Group for Management of Fluid Distension Media in Operative Hysteroscopy. 2016.

6. Vachharajani TJ, Zaman F, Abreo KD Hyponatremia in critically ill patients. J Intensive Care Med 2003;18:3–8.

7. Verbalis JG, Goldsmith SR,Greenberg A, Korzelius C,Schrier RW, Sterns RH, Thompson CJ Diagnosis, evaluation, and treatment of hyponatremia: expert panel recommendations. Am J Med 2013;126(10):S1–S42.

Index